HOMEOPATHY
911

HOMEOPATHY
911

What to Do in an
EMERGENCY
Before Help Arrives

**Eileen Nauman, D.H.M. (UK), EMT-B
with Gail Derin-Kellogg, O.M.D., EMT-B**

KENSINGTON BOOKS
http://www.kensingtonbooks.com

KENSINGTON BOOKS are published by

Kensington Publishing Corp.
850 Third Avenue
New York, NY 10022

ISBN 1-57566-694-4

First Kensington Trade Paperback Printing: July, 2000
10 9 8 7 6 5 4 3 2 1

Printed in the United States of America

To my husband, Dave Nauman,
my mother, Ruth Gent and to my
incredible editor, Claire Gerus—
thank you for all your help, support and guidance,

and

To the mother, father, husband or wife
who has been caught in an emergency
situation and felt helpless, not knowing how
to respond or what to do,

May this book and the knowledge
contained in it, help save lives.

CONTENTS

FOREWORD

Edward Kondrot, MD

Emergency! Trauma! Injury! Even the most seasoned practitioner will panic and draw a blank during this time. Eileen and Gail have written a superb reference book that will help us when faced with an emergency situation with precious little time to react.

Homeopaths are in a unique position to assist the vital force in these times of crisis and in many cases have the opportunity to change the outcome before emergency help arrives. This book will make it easy for us to mobilize our remedies in times of crisis.

This reference book is well written and indexed for a rapid location of any emergency situation. In the table of contents, emergencies are listed A through Z for very easy access. Each emergency is organized by definition, signs, symptoms, and indicators, along with emergency medical and homeopathic treatment. One can quickly locate the emergency and immediately have a practical emergency treatment plan.

There is also a materia medica, which is an excellent reference source. When these situations present themselves, you no longer will call 911 and wonder what else can be done. This book will help all of us, professional or lay practitioners, to take the necessary life-saving steps. This book will make a big difference in the management of emergencies.

Jack Forbush, RN, CCRN, CEN

Having spent the last decade devoted to providing emergency medical care, I have learned to appreciate the great need for educating the general public, particularly in rural areas.

Oftentimes, definitive emergency care is delayed due to extended distances, environmental issues, and in some areas inadequate emergency services. Organizations such as the American Heart Association and the American Red Cross have moved mountains in their efforts to remedy this dilemma through public education in CPR and first aid procedures. *Help!* and *Homeopathy* expands this knowledge base for the lay homeopathic community by providing a solid first-line arsenal of homeopathic remedies.

This book is an incredible undertaking. The enormous time and effort required to compile a reference source for both the lay person and practitioner is astonishing. Many will find this book immensely useful. It provides a general overview of accepted first aid techniques while interjecting advanced topics for the practitioner. As a parallel to this information, *Help!* and *Homeopathy* provides references to remedies applicable to the emergency situation.

My sincere thanks and appreciation to Eileen, Gail, and all those involved in providing us with such a resourceful text.

ACKNOWLEDGMENTS

Without the help of Rosemarie Brown, MSW, DIHom (UK), EMT, and Gail Derin-Kellogg, OMD, EMT, this book would not have come about. Thanks to Captain Jerry Doerksin, Cottonwood Fire Department and paramedic, who was our EMT instructor at Yavapai College, Cottonwood, Arizona. He good naturedly put up with three homeopaths in his class. And to Mary Buckner, RN, who was a great set of eyes on this project, as well.

Our thanks extends to Ed Kondrot, M.D. and Jack Forbush, RN and paramedic, both homeopaths, who have given their time, care, and love to our vision contained within this book. And last, but never least, to Julian Winston, one of the truest friends that homeopathy in the United States has ever had, for his keen eye, discernment, enthusiasm, and help. This book has many creators. And we are grateful to all of you. Thank you.

INTRODUCTION

When Gail and I took an Emergency Medical Technician course from Yavapai College in Cottonwood, Arizona, we had to write down all of our life-saving procedures, along with what was known collectively as "SSI's"—signs, symptoms and indicators—of specific emergencies that a baby, child, or adult might have. The EMT had to know these and be able to make a call on them, out in the field, and patch through to the emergency room of the nearest hospital as the individual was transported as quickly as possible for medical help.

As a homeopath for 27 years, I was struck by the number of times that a specific homeopathic remedy could also work in tandem, right alongside these EMT lifesaving procedures, and it would support these ongoing activities even more. And so this book was born, to meld together two different types of medical application into one book in the hope that it might save a life, or add a little time to that 'golden hour' during transit to the nearest medical facility.

So many of our emergencies occur at home. And it would be nice to have a book where such procedures were available in plain English, alphabetized by name, with a list of what to do. That is the reason for this book. **It does not take the place of the 911 call.** Indeed, the FIRST thing you need to do if there is an accident, and if someone is at home who can help, is send them to call 911 while you care for the injured victim. Or, if you're home alone, make the 911 call first and then go help the victim.

Every home, as far as I'm concerned, should have a homeopathic first aid kit. One is available that goes with this book. It is known as the Advanced First Aid Kit and it can be purchased directly from Hahnemann Homeopathic Pharmacy, San Rafael, California. Please look in Appendix A for more information.

Secondly, it is vital that you have established a relationship with a homeopathic practitioner in your own area. If you do not have a homeopath, please go to Appendix C where information on how to find a homeopath is provided. If you have a family homeopath, it is important to have a talk about emergencies around your home. Many times a homeopath may want the parents to have a higher potency of a specific remedy on hand, such as a 200C or 1M. If you are not a professional, you should NEVER use a potency higher than 30C. Your homeopath may give you specific instructions to carry out in case of a specific emergency—do that. Use this book as an adjunct, a guide, and a place to start a discussion with your homeopath, who may have differences of opinion on a remedy for a specific condition. Your homeopath's final word should be used in lieu of the remedy in this book as they will know the constitutional remedy for the members of your family. Always consult with your homeopath and talk over emergency situations, what procedures to take, and in what order.

After making the 911 call, your next focus should be on your injured family member. After emergency help arrives, give your homeopath a call.

Every home should have parents who are certified by the American Heart Association for CPR, trained in the Heimlich Maneuver, and trained in first aid, as well. Armed with these three procedures, lives can quite literally be saved. Should they get into a medical emergency, your children stand a far greater chance of surviving it than if you didn't know the above procedures. Another very important phone number to always have in a very readable place is the Poison Control number for your state. Have your fire department/ambulance number, police/sheriff number, hospital emergency room number, and your child's doctor's number all readily available. You do not want to have to search because each minute can count toward living or dying. It is important to keep these numbers near the phone where they are quickly accessible.

A list of emergency supplies you should have on hand can be found in Appendix B.

It is our hope that this book helps to save lives via emergency procedure guidelines as well as homeopathically.

PUBLISHER'S NOTE

This book is not intended to take the place of qualified help in an emergency—either medical or homeopathic. In any emergency, call or send for help immediately. This book is meant to provide life-saving procedures when qualified help may take some time to arrive. It is recommended that you take a certified CPR and first aid course and learn the Heimlich Maneuver. If possible, always have protective equipment in your home or car which consists of latex or vinyl gloves and a mouth barrier with a one-way valve.

The author and publisher of this book have made certain that all medical techniques and references are correct and compatible with the national standards generally accepted at the time of publication. The author and publisher disclaim any liability, loss, injury or damage incurred as a consequence, directly or indirectly, of the use and application of the contents of this book.

IMPORTANT: The procedures described in this book are based upon and follow the American Heart Association guidelines for Basic Life Support.

TRANSMISSION OF AIDS AND HEPATITIS B VIRUS: Anyone responding to an emergency should be guided by moral and ethical values of preserving life. In responding to an emergency, do what you think/feel is best. The American Heart Association notes that if you are in doubt about exposure to the above viruses (especially with someone you do not know who is not a family member), and won't initiate mouth-to-mouth ventilation (CPR procedures), then call for an ambulance, open the airway, skip rescue breathing (mouth to mouth), and do chest compressions. If possible, always have latex or vinyl gloves on your person, in your car glove box or somewhere handy at home.

ABOUT THE AUTHORS

Eileen Nauman, DHM, DIHom (UK), EMT, is a classically trained homeopath who has practiced for thirty years. A graduate of the British Institute of Homeopathy in England, she is a member of their faculty. She is on the core faculty of the Desert Institute of Classical Homeopathy, Phoenix, Arizona.

Moderator and owner of http://www.medicinegarden.com, an Internet web site that includes alternative medicine and an active mailing list, she creates a classroom atmosphere to teach people introductory homeopathy, and shows how they can use it to help themselves, their families, and their pets.

Eileen has lectured around the world on various alternative medicine techniques, including classical homeopathy, emergency medicine and homeopathy, and flower and gem essences,

She is the author of Poisons That Heal (Light Technology, Sedona, AZ, 1995), a book on homeopathy and epidemics, and is a contributing author in CLINICIAN'S COMPLETE REFERENCE TO COMPLEMENTARY MEDICINE by Donald Novey, MD (Mosby Publishing, February, 2000). She provided information on homeopathy, flower and gem essences, Native American healing and quartz crystal healing. She is currently working on Beauty in Bloom: Homeopathy for Menopause (Blue Turtle Publishing, Cottonwood, AZ, May, 2000).

P.O. Box 2513
Cottonwood, AZ 86326
Internet web site: http://www.medicinegarden.com
Alternative medicine list: athena@medicinegarden.com
E-mail: docbones@sedona.net

Gail Derin is a nationally certified EMT and a Doctor of Oriental Medicine. Gail is a classically trained homeopath. She is a graduate of Hahnemann Homeopathic College, Albany, California. Some of her focus has been working with post-traumatic stress syndrome (PTSD) with Vietnam Vets using homeopathy. She has been in practice for seventeen years; she also instructs martial arts to provide health through body and mind.

E-mail: gailbruc@discoverynet.com

Chapter 1

HOW TO USE THIS BOOK

When an emergency strikes at home, in the car, on vacation, or out hiking, your mind can go right out the window. In a crisis, emergency phone numbers should be somewhere handy and easy to find. There are times when 911 is not available or you are too far away from a phone. Or, you have a cell phone, but 911 response can be 30 to 60 minutes away—which cuts into the 'golden hour' where lives teeter in the balance between medical help and what you can do to help in the meantime. That is the purpose of this book.

After making the 911 call, it can be equally lifesaving to be able to get to one source that has lifesaving information in it to help you until the proper medical help can arrive on the scene.

This book is arranged alphabetically to be flipped through and read quickly to find out what to do. Always follow the Emergency Medical Response guidelines. These are based upon the American Heart Association and Emergency Medical Technician recommendations.

Your next step will be to administer the correct homeopathic remedy. Hopefully you have a family homeopath with whom you can discuss the remedies in this book before any emergencies arise. If you do not, the remedies are guidelines for AFTER you have taken the appropriate medical emergency steps.

This book provides a bridge to utilizing homeopathy during an emergency situation; but it is always best to have first consulted a homeopath in your town or city.

What Is Homeopathy?

Homeopathy is a system of medicine developed in Germany by Dr. Samuel Hahnemann more than 200 years ago. Since that time, it has spread to every country of the world. Homeopathy is based on the Law of Similars, or 'like cures like'. This means that, while a substance given in large dosages will produce specific symptoms, when reduced in size and administered in very tiny doses, it will stimulate the body's reactive processes to remove these symptoms. For example, Ipecac if taken in large quantity, will produce vomiting. Yet, when taken in minute doses, it cures vomiting. In addition, homeopathy is very safe—it is almost impossible to overdose on a remedy.

1

How to Find the Correct Homeopathic Remedy

To get the right remedy, you must match the symptoms of the person with the symptoms of the remedies that are available for the specific injury. After locating your emergency in the EMERGENCIES A-Z section, you will see a selection of remedies. Go to Chapter 4, page 159, and check each remedy. When you find one with three or more matching symptoms with those of the injured person, use the remedy.

Dosage and Potency Instructions

This book has been set up to respond to emergencies after they have occurred and BEFORE trained medical help (EMTs or paramedics) can arrive to take over the scene with lifesaving equipment. Generally speaking, if you live in a city, 911 help may be 5 to 15 minutes, maximum, away from you. If you live out in the country, it may be 15 minutes to an hour before qualified medical help can arrive.

What you do for the injured person between the 911 call and their arrival is paramount. You may save a person's life, or at the least, stabilize them by knowing what to do and what not to do in the meantime.

Strictly follow the dosage guidelines. NEVER exceed the dosages recommended in this book. Many times, the injured person is semiconscious or unconscious. NEVER put dry pellets of a homeopathic remedy in their mouth. The skin is able to absorb a remedy. Use the fluid method of delivering a homeopathic remedy. They are known as *dilutions*. See Appendix E, page 216, on how to make a dilution from pellet form.

How to Apply a Homeopathic Dilution

♦ **If the person is semiconscious or unconscious:**

Place one drop of the chosen remedy dilution onto the underside of the person's wrist and rub it in. If impossible to put on wrist, put a drop behind the ear, where the skin is very thin, as it is in the wrist area.

When you do this, do NOT rub vigorously (in case head or spinal injuries are present). GENTLY apply it in a circular motion to an area about the size of a dime. One drop only. You do not need more. Then follow the directions in this book on how often and how many times you should reapply the dilution.

♦ **If the person is fully conscious:**

If the person is fully conscious and there are NO problems with their airway or breathing, hold the open bottle close to their nostrils and have them breathe in. This is known as "olfaction." If their symptoms do not change within 10 minutes, then place ONE drop of the dilution beneath their tongue. If they begin to become semiconscious or you see alternating states of consciousness, apply one drop to the underside of their wrist or directly behind the ear per dosage instructions above.

It is always SAFER to apply to their skin than into their mouth if there's any question as to whether or not they are fully conscious. In emergency situations, people who are injured can panic and go into shock—and this can happen so suddenly, that giving a drop by mouth may exacerbate your problems and not help the person or you.

TO BE ON THE SAFE SIDE, APPLY ONE DROP TO THE UNDERSIDE OF THE WRIST EVERY 15 MINUTES.

♦ **What if the person is unconscious and I do not have dilutions, but only dry pellets, instead? Should I give these white homeopathic pills, by dropping them into the mouth?**

No! If they are unconscious, do NOT put these pills or dilution drops into their mouth—they may go down the windpipe and create even more problems for the person later on.

Instead, always carry a one-ounce eye dropper bottle filled with brandy. In an emergency situation, you can drop 10 to 20 pellets of the remedy into the bottle, cap it, shake it for a minute and then do the following: Using the eye dropper, place ONE drop on the inside of the person's wrist or directly behind their ear. Rub the drop into the person's skin. The skin will absorb the homeopathic remedy. Do this every 15 minutes until help arrives, or until the symptoms stop, or up to six dosages, whichever occurs first.

In this way, you will not choke or cause more problems for the person. Never, ever put these pellets into an unconscious person's mouth. Always rub it on the inside of their wrist or behind their ear.

♦ **If the person's symptoms go away—do not give any more of the homeopathic dilution.**

Homeopathic remedies are the opposite of traditional drug-type medications. If the injured person's symptoms go away after one application of the homeopathic dilution, do NOT give the remedy again, but WAIT.

If the symptoms start to reappear, then rub another drop on the underside of the person's wrist.

Generally speaking, 911 help will arrive within the allotted time of six doses outlined in this book, given 15 minutes apart. That is an hour and a half—plenty of time to get professional medical care.

♦ **What if I'm out in the woods, 50 miles away from a hospital?**

There are many answers to this question and none of them may cover your particular emergency situation. Much depends upon if you are with a third person (besides the injured party) or not. One can remain with the injured person while one of you hikes out for medical help.

If it is only you and the injured party, your next question is whether they are conscious, semiconscious, experiencing altered levels of consciousness, or unconscious. If conscious, do what you can as outlined in this book, and they can apply the drop of the remedy into their own mouths. One drop beneath the tongue, and then every 15 minutes thereafter. If their symptoms are still there but are diminished by taking the homeopathic remedy, they can continue to dose themselves until the symptoms are gone.

The normal dosage is SIX times. However, a situation like this calls for a different plan. Generally speaking, most people can take up to 12 doses of a 30C potency homeopathic remedy before 'proving' it.

A 'proving' occurs when the maximum amount of dosages has been taken by the injured person and the symptoms that were going away or were stabilized start to COME BACK. This is not a good situation to find oneself in—so dosage must be carefully counted and respected.

FOR EXAMPLE: If the remedy halted most of the bleeding, and if the injured person continues to take the remedy every 15 minutes and exceeds the 12-dose limit, the bleeding can begin again—which is not good. After a maximum of 12 doses, follow the steps below.

♦ **Here's what to do if you must go beyond 12 doses:**

Providing the person is conscious or you've got a third party who can perform this function for the injured person, take the dilution bottle into your hand:

1. Open the palm of your left hand.

2. With your right hand, strike the bottom of the remedy against your left, open palm with a strong, jarring motion. Do this 100 times. This is called 'succussion.' It moves the remedy up one potency from what it was originally, from a 30C to a higher resolution. This will hopefully avoid PROVING problems until medical help can arrive. This is called 'plussing.'

3. Then, give the remedy to the person—one drop. Wait 15 minutes.

4.   The next time, if you must give the remedy again, do the same thing: Succuss the remedy 100 times in the palm of your hand. You now have a 32C of the remedy. Give one drop and wait 15 minutes. If the symptoms begin to return:

5.   Succuss the remedy 100 more times in the palm of your hand. You now have a 33C of the remedy. Give one drop and wait 15 minutes.

6.   You may continue to do this until medical help arrives—BUT—if the 'old' original symptoms begin to come back, STOP GIVING THE REMEDY. Do what you can with the information outlined in this book for emergency medical response, only.

Contacting Your Family Homeopath

Contact your family homeopath as soon as you can after calling 911 and seeing that the injured person is taken care of as best you can. Do NOT run to call the homeopath if the injured person needs your help. WAIT until AFTER 911 help has arrived and you've answered any questions that they might have. Then call your homeopath.

Some homeopaths work closely with their patients and may already have 'trained' you in many general family emergency situations that can occur. Some do not. It is a good idea to consult with your homeopath on emergency situations—before they happen—so you both know what is expected of the other. If you have not, then it is time to do it.

It is important to contact your homeopath, especially if the injured person is their patient. They can prescribe another remedy or give you information about the remedy you are using, and what to do after the injured person is in the emergency room of the hospital. They may give you different dosage instructions—follow them. They also carry higher potencies and know how to dispense them and are trained in this area, where you are not. NEVER use any potency higher than a 30C without the express permission and guidance from your homeopath first.

During an emergency, homeopathic medicine can be an equal lifesaver to what you do medically for the injured person.

What If I Don't Have a Family Homeopath?

You can call the National Center for Homeopathy in Alexandria, Virginia, and purchase, for a minimal price, a U.S. directory of practicing homeopaths. It lists the homeopaths by state. Call 1-703-548-7790. Or, if you are on the Internet, the directory is free at http://www.healthy.net. Or, http://www.dimensional/~SteveW. You can also e-mail them at nchinfo@igc.apc.org for more information on homeopathy.

Other Questions

♦ **I see you recommend a 30C potency. Why is that?**

It is generally accepted in the United States that 30C is a 'safe' potency to sell over the counter to people who want to utilize homeopathy. The truth is that 30C is often considered quite a high potency that can, if taken too many times, cause a 'proving' in a person. A proving means all the old symptoms that you were trying to get rid of will come back. That is why the maximum dosage for any remedy in this book is SIX. To give more than six doses is to potentially create a proving in a sensitive person. And you do not want this on top of everything else that you are dealing with during an emergency.

If it is the right potency, then it should be curative. If it is the wrong one, you may see a proving. And, generally speaking, with three doses of the correct remedy you will see dramatic results. In some cases, even the 'right' remedy isn't going to fix the situation, such as in the case of a severe hemorrhage. The right remedy, along with direct or indirect pressure, will slow the bleeding considerably. That is what you are looking for in the 'right' remedy—a lessening, but not disappearance, of a certain symptom. Surgery may be the only long-term way to permanently fix or cure the wound or situation.

However, if you are out in the middle of nowhere, you can use succussion (see previous page), and hopefully will avoid a proving situation. Sometimes this is possible and other times it is not. In cases where it is not, you must STOP giving the remedy immediately.

♦ **If my homeopath gives me a higher potency and tells me to use it instead of what is in your book, what should I do?**

Follow the recommendations of your homeopath—always. The potency and dosages in this book are guidelines, not absolutes. It is best if you are under the care of a homeopath to take this book to them and discuss it thoroughly, ahead of time. That way, if there is an emergency, your homeopath may have already given you a different remedy or a remedy of higher potency to use instead—and you can have crossed out what is in this book and written in his or her instructions and recommendations instead.

◆ **I see that throughout your book you never recommend more than six doses of a remedy. Why?**

Because in a sensitive individual, over six administrations of a 30C potency of any remedy can create a 'proving'. This means that the old symptoms the person had will come back—and other symptoms may also appear that the person did not have that are associated with the remedy.

Your best course of action is this: When the symptoms stop, stop taking the remedy—or succuss it (for instructions on how to do that, see page 4).

◆ **Are homeopathic remedies like drugs I get from my doctor? Do I have to take so many every so many hours?**

Absolutely not! Homeopathic remedies are just the OPPOSITE of traditional medical drugs. Generally speaking, in non-emergency situations, you take one remedy, one time, and then wait—and your symptoms go away.

In an emergency situation, you may have to dose more frequently—every 15 minutes—or more frequently before the symptoms will subside or go away. If the injured person's symptoms go away, do NOT give another dose. If the symptoms start coming back, give a second dose, and so on. Once the symptoms are gone—do nothing else homeopathically—no more dosing. You may well need more than one dose—but never go over six. Generally speaking, professional medical help has arrived within this time frame and usually you will have given only one or two doses, maximum, before they arrive, which is fine.

◆ **After professional medical help arrives, should I still dose the injured person with the homeopathic remedy?**

No. Let the paramedics or EMTs do their job. If you are the parent of the child or a spouse, you can ride along in the ambulance with them. At this phase, bring your remedies and the book with you—and at the hospital, if you have a family homeopath, call them and ask what to do next. Tell the homeopath what remedy you gave, what potency, and how many times you administered it. They will then have a plan of action to continue with after that.

◆ **What if I'm not close to a phone to call 911?**

Then follow the procedures outlined in this book and if you have your homeopathic kit with you, check out the remedy symptoms against the person's symptoms. If they match closely (it does not have to be 100%), follow the dosage guidelines. Six doses at 15 minutes apart gives you time, hopefully, to find the help you need. That is one and a half hours. If this is a life-threatening emergency, the 'golden hour' rule is in force, anyway.

♦ **What about an unconscious baby? How should I administer the homeopathic remedy?**

The same way you would for a semiconscious, alternating states, or unconscious adult—see page 2. Just place a drop on the inside of the baby's wrist or behind the ear, and GENTLY rub it in.

♦ **If the symptoms stop in the injured person, I stop giving the homeopathic remedy, right?**

Right! If the symptoms go away, do NOT re-dose the person. However, if the symptoms start to come back, give them the next dose—up to six doses.

♦ **What will the EMTs or paramedics think of me giving a homeopathic remedy?**

In all likelihood, they may never have heard of homeopathy, although that is changing. It is important, if they ask you if the injured person has taken anything, to tell them what was given homeopathically. If time is of the essence, you won't be going into a long, detailed explanation anyway—you can save that for later, and explain if necessary.

Explain to them that these are not drugs because professionals in the medical service need to know what traditional medical drugs the person is on presently or has been given.

You can tell the professionals that the homeopathy in no way interferes, and that it works naturally with the body's systems and organs to help cure the problem the injured person presently has. They need to be reassured that the homeopathy does not interfere—and it does not. It can only help in such a situation.

♦ **Does homeopathy work poorly with traditional drugs?**

Yes and no. Homeopathy can work in tandem with traditional medical drugs. Traditional drugs will slow down the effects or may antidote the homeopathic remedy on the person. There are no adverse side effects or contraindications from giving traditional drugs (such as pain killers) after you've taken a homeopathic remedy. You may, under the guidance of your homeopath, have to administer the remedy.

Chapter 2

HOW TO EXAMINE A PERSON

One of the most important things you will do after an accident or injury is to perform a primary survey on the person. When adrenaline is pumping, we all tend to blank out, we might get far more emotional than normal, or we can't think of what to do next. The examination technique described below can save a life after you have called 911. Known as a Primary Survey, it is designed to identify life-threatening conditions.

This book assumes you already have CPR and Heimlich training.

"Universal Protection"

Nowadays, sadly, there is great potential danger for a good samaritan such as yourself to contract deadly or serious blood-transmissible ailments if you help an injured person. AIDS, HIV, and Hepatitis B are all transmitted via body fluids.

It is wise to always carry a set of latex or vinyl protective gloves with you, in your car glove box, in ' our hiking pack, or wherever you go that you might encounter an accident.

Many people are allergic to latex, but there are non-latex gloves available for you. Protective gloves can be bought at any medical outlet. I would advise a thicker, heavier pair rather than sheer, thin latex because you do not know what that injured person may have and the thicker, better quality of glove stops viral and bacterial transmission much better than the thinner, cheaper type. In this case, it will be money well spent on a good pair of protectiv gloves.

Because of the threat of contracting a horrendous disease out of your goodness of heart to help someone at an accident scene, it is up to you whether or not you give CPR or anything else if you do not have protective gloves with you. It is up to the individual. **Is the scene safe? Make sure it is.**

The Initial Survey

With that in mind, let's look at how to go about performing the A, B, C's of the Primary Survey. This is also, on occasion, known as the "15-Second Global" where speed and time are critical and one does not have time to tarry due to the nature of the person's injuries.

♦ **Remember: "Universal Protection"—Put Those Gloves on Before You Touch the Injured Person!!!!**

"A" = **Airway**. Try to arouse the person by touching their shoulder and speaking to them. Do not shake them unnecessarily as they may have a spinal cord injury. "Hey, you okay? Can you hear me?" If they do not respond … according to CPR measures, you are to shout to someone to call 911 as you move forward with CPR management. However, if the person is conscious, then …

"B" = **Breathing**. "Look, listen, and feel" for breathing. Look toward their chest. Lean over the person with your ear very close to their nose and mouth. Do you hear anything? Does the person have an adequate airway in order to breathe? Is the person having difficulty breathing? Is their breathing shallow, deep, making snoring sounds, rapid, or normal? Are they choking on something? Look inside their mouth and see if their dental plate has clogged their airway. Or is a broken tooth or teeth jammed back down in their throat preventing them from breathing? Or is there mucus? Blood? Or other debris in their mouth? Is the person's skin turning blue around their mouth or their fingernail beds (cyanotic)? If they aren't breathing begin CPR management. If the person is CONSCIOUS and BREATHING …

"C" = **Circulation**. You will assess their pulse to see whether or not the blood is reaching all areas of the body. Using two fingers, check their radial pulse on the underside of their wrist, just below their thumb. If absent, check the other wrist. If there is none, go to the carotid artery on the side of their neck. Press gently and only one side at a time. Note if pulse is thready, bounding, soft, or full (see Glossary). If pulse is not present, go to CPR management.

a. If pulse is present, assess the person's skin color and tone. Are they pale, waxy looking, skin marbleized with veins showing, mottled, bluish, red and flushed, or purple looking? All are indicators of shock. Bluish skin indicates cyanosis or lack of oxygen.

b. Is the skin clammy, or wet? This is a sign of shock.

c. Check temperature and moisture by touching their skin. Is it hot? Feverish? Chilled? There may be fever (heat in skin) or shock (cool, clammy, cold skin). Hot and dry skin could be a sign of heat stroke.

d. Perform a Capillary Refill ("cap refill") on their thumbnail. Place their thumb between your thumb and index finger. Place firm, downward pressure on their nailbed and quickly release it. The nailbed will turn white as you press on it—you are pressing the capillary blood out of that immediate region. As you release the nailbed, the blood flow should return to that nailbed in TWO SECONDS or less. If it does not, this is an indicator of impaired circulation. Treat for shock.

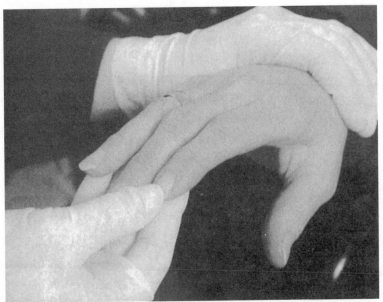

As a final check of the patient's circulatory status, assess the capillary refill (photo reprinted with permission from the American Academy of Orthopaedic Surgeons).

e. Perform a quick scan for obvious bleeding and its control. The major pulse points of the body are shown in the figure on the next page. Pressure on either the **brachial** or **femoral** artery points **ONLY** with the heel of your hand can slow bleeding considerably. NEVER use that kind of pressure on the carotid arteries.

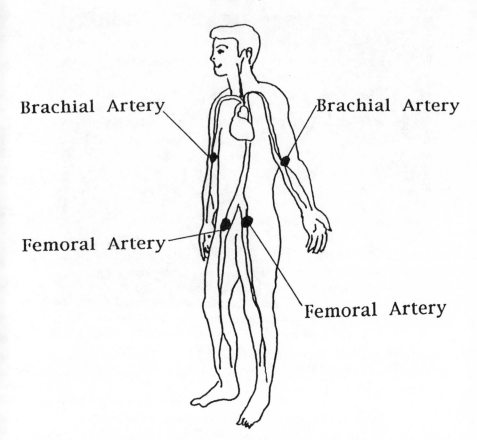

Brachial Artery

Brachial Artery

Femoral Artery

Femoral Artery

Major arterial pulse points to use to stop bleeding below that particular site (illustration courtesy of the American Academy of Orthopaedic Surgeons).

Secondary Examination of a Person

After you are assured they have an open airway, and they are breathing adequately and their circulation is not impaired, you can begin the next step of your examination. You can always ask them: "Where do you hurt?" Or, "Where's the pain?" Be in communication with them at all times. Just because they tell you the pain is "here" does not mean you do not perform your examination—you do—and you do it on the front of their body and the back of their body (examine the back ONLY if absolutely necessary because they may have a spinal injury and you do NOT want to move them).

Generally speaking, if you have done the A, B, C's, by then the 911 medical responders have probably already arrived or are just about to. You need not perform a secondary survey because they will. Stand aside and let them work, but be sure to tell them your assessments, too. They may prove to be vital pieces of information.

In another scenario, where 911 isn't going to arrive for 15 to 30 minutes, a secondary survey is a must because you have to understand the extent of the person's injury(s) to help them survive until medical help arrives. It is with this scenario that what is written below should be undertaken by yourself or your partner. Start with their head and work down to their toes.

♦ **Remember Universal Protection—Put Those Gloves On!!!**

HEAD: Run your fingers lightly through their hair and check their entire scalp. Feel for deformity, swelling, or bleeding. If yes, see Head Injuries, page 99 and Shock, page 140.

EARS: Check behind their ears (look for Battle's sign—bruising of the mastoid process which would indicate head injury), look IN their ears for fluids or blood, check their brow. If yes, see Head Injuries, page 99 and Shock, page 140.

EYES: Look at their eyes (do they have a black eye? Sign of a head injury. Blood in eyes? Impaled object in eye?) Look in their eyes for fluids leaking from the corners of them; look at the pupil size. (Are they equal or unequal? If unequal, this indicates a head injury.) If yes, see Head Injury, page 99, Eye Injury, page 86, and Shock, page 140.

NOSE: Check their nostrils. (Any fluid coming out of them? What kind? If pink or clear, possibly spinal fluid escaping, indicating serious head injury.) If blood, it can still indicate a serious head injury. If yes, see Head Injury, page 99 and Shock, page 140.

MOUTH: Check in their mouth. (Dentures loose? A tooth loose in the mouth? Is it lodged or lying in the rear of their throat causing breathing problems? Any objects in their mouth or rear of their throat? Is there blood, vomitus, or fluid collecting in the mouth?) If yes, see Soft Tissue Injuries, page 147 and Shock, page 140.

NECK/REAR OF SKULL: Palpate very gently and thoroughly the back of the neck (without moving it) and feel for any 'step-outs' or vertebrae sticking out of line from the spinal column in an odd or unusual position. If so, be sure to maintain the present position of the neck to prevent further movement. Feel the base of the skull for any swelling, deformity, or bleeding. Palpate the sides and front of the neck looking for swelling, bruising, or deformity. If yes, see Spinal Injury, page 149 and Shock, page 140.

CHEST/ARMS/HANDS: With hands open, and with three fingers of each hand, press gently down upon the collarbones and move out toward their shoulders. Continue firm pressing. Do you feel crepitus? This is the grinding of bones that are broken. Or if you feel a crackling, bubbling feeling beneath the skin, this is subcutaneous emphysema. Are there any deformities? Place your hands on their shoulders and press inward. Any crepitus? With both hands, squeeze each arm gently, feeling for deformities, swelling, or bleeding, down to their fingers. With hands open, press against the upper chest and see if the breastbone is broken or if ribs are broken. Placing hands on either side of the rib cage, press IN. Any crepitus? If yes, see Chest Injuries, page 49 and Shock, page 140

ABDOMEN: Divide the abdomen into four quadrants using the belly button as the center of this arrangement. Mentally draw a vertical line from the end of the breastbone down to above the person's pelvic bone. Then mentally draw a horizontal line right through the center of the belly button to each side of the person. These are the four quadrants.

With three fingers, palpate the upper right quadrant (above the belly button and to the person's right), then palpate the upper left quadrant (above the belly button and to the person's left), palpate the lower right quadrant (below the belly button and to the person's right) and palpate the lower left quadrant (below the belly button and the person's left). Feel for tenderness or any unusual hardness or swelling in any of these areas. If yes, see Abdominal Injury, page 21 and Shock, page 140.

HIPS: Press IN on both hips with your hands. Any crepitus? Gently press down on the tops of the hip region. Any crepitus? Gently press down with the heel of one of your hands on the pubis or just above the crotch area. Any crepitus? If yes, see Dislocation, page 69, Fracture, page 94, and Shock, page 140.

THIGHS: Use both hands and firmly feel all around the thighs. Look for deformity, hardness, and swelling. If yes, see Fracture, page 94 and Shock, page 140.

KNEES: Use both hands and feel for any deformity, swelling, or hardness. If yes, see Fracture, page 94, Shock, page 140, and Soft Tissue Injuries, page 149.

CALVES/ANKLES: Use both hands and feel for any deformity, swelling or hardness. If yes, see Fracture, page 94, Shock, page 140, and Soft Tissue Injuries, page 149.

FEET: Use both hands and feel for any deformity, swelling, or hardness. If yes, see Fracture, page 94, Shock, page 140, and Soft Tissue Injuries, page 149.

You have now completed a frontal survey. Unless you are out where there is no 911 or medical help coming, you should NOT move the person to check the rear of them unless you are assured there is no spinal injury. If you see blood leaking out from beneath them, then you must perform a "log roll" and turn them from their back, and onto their side to examine the back of their head, their entire back, buttocks, and thigh region.

Here's how to perform a log roll, which will give your injured person maximum protection against a possible spinal injury:

How to Perform a Log Roll On an Injured Person

1. You need at least two people to do this. If you have three people, that is best.

2. One person stabilizes the head and neck with both hands. Place your hands on the sides of their jaw, with your fingers stretched downward to cradle the neck simultaneously. This is to stabilize the neck so it will not turn or twist. It if does, it can mean more spinal injury. The person who is maintaining support of the person's head and neck will be responsible to verbally count out loud to "three." On her count, the other two people will turn the injured person from their back onto their side (the uninjured side). The person is always rolled TOWARD you on her count.

3. The second person positions one of his hands on the injured person's shoulder and the other one on the hip.

4. If there is a third person, they would place one hand on the buttocks/hip area and one on the calves/ankles of the person.

5. At the count of "three"—given by the person holding the injured person's head and neck in place—roll the person TOWARD you onto their uninjured side.

6. One of the two people kneeling alongside the injured person would then do a 'sweep' of the back of their head, neck, back, hips, buttocks, and legs. If anything was found, it should be noted or appropriately cared for.

7. Once the sweep is done, at the count of "three" by the person holding the head of the injured person, simultaneously roll the person onto their back once again. If available, place a blanket beneath them.

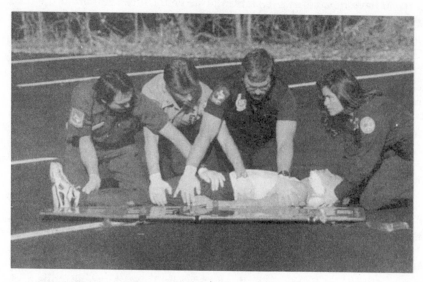

The rescuer supporting the head and cervical spine is responsible for coordinating the log-roll procedure through direct, verbal commands. Positioning the hands on the far side of the patient increases leverage for the rescuers. Weight control is best achieved through a smooth, coordinated pull using the rescuers' body weight and their shoulder and back muscles. The rescuers should concentrate their pull on the heavier portions of the patient's body. (Photo reprinted with permission from the American Academy of Orthopaedic Surgeons.)

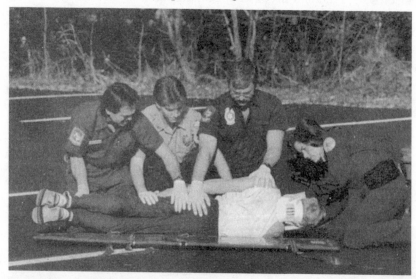

♦ **Assessing neurals in a possible spinal cord injury:**
Ask the person if there are any areas where they feel tingling, weakness, or numbness. Ask them to wriggle their fingers and toes. Ask them to hold out their hands (if possible) and try to resist as you **gently** push down on them. Then, place your hands beneath their palms and ask them to try to resist as you **gently** push upward—see if there is any strength in the person's response. Ask them to squeeze your fingers with their hands. If they cannot do one of these, this indicates a possible spinal injury. Touch the inside and outside of their leg and ask them which leg you are touching, and which side of their leg is being touched. If they do not answer correctly, this also confirms spinal cord injury.

♦ **Modified jaw thrust:**
This technique is used when neck and spinal injury is suspected. Do not try to perform CPR the routine way you have been taught if the person has neck injuries. To lift or change the position of the neck might cause further damage. Instead, use a modified jaw thrust as shown in the following photos. Kneel behind the person's head. Place your fingers behind the angle of the person's jaw and gently and firmly bring it forward (keeping in mind that you are NOT moving the neck). Then, use your index and long fingers to hold the jaw in that forward position, while simultaneously compressing the person's nose with your thumbs (so air cannot escape). CPR can then be rendered mouth-to-mouth without moving the neck.

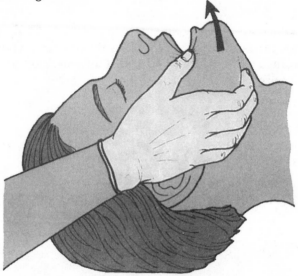

In the jaw-thrust maneuver, place your fingers behind the angle of the patient's jaw and forcefully bring it forward.

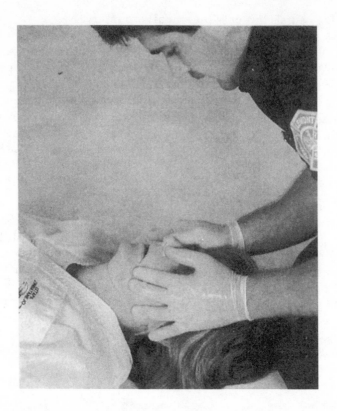

The modified jaw-thrust maneuver. Use the index and long fingers to thrust the jaw forward while you compress the nose with your thumbs. (Photo reprinted with permission from the American Academy of Orthopaedic Surgeons.)

Chapter 3

EMERGENCIES A THROUGH Z

★ABDOMINAL EVISCERATION★

DEFINITION: A wound to the abdomen where the intestines are exposed to the open air. The intestines must be kept moist under all conditions; the tissues will be destroyed if they are allowed to dry out. Also referred to as one's "guts hanging out."

TREATMENT:

EMERGENCY MEDICAL RESPONSE:

1. Place a compress that is MOIST over the area. Do NOT place any material that clings or loses its substance when wet—no toilet paper, facial tissue, absorbent cotton, or paper towels on the intestines. Do **not** attempt to push the organs back into the abdomen.
2. Seal this dressing with aluminum foil or plastic on top of it, taped on all four sides to uninjured abdominal skin. This will keep the organs moist and warm.
3. Treat for Shock, page 140.

HOMEOPATHIC:

1. **Arnica Montana 30C,** one dose every 15 minutes to halt hemorrhaging. Up to six doses.
2. **China 30C,** one dose every 15 minutes. Up to six doses.
3. **Phosphorus 30C,** one dose every 15 minutes. Up to six doses.
4. **Carbo Vegetabilis 30C,** one dose every 15 minutes. Up to six doses.

NOTES _____

_____

_____

_____

_____

★ABDOMINAL INJURY★

DEFINITION: A common injury when a driver strikes the steering wheel in an accident (and is not wearing a seat belt or is wearing the seat belt too low or incorrectly). Bruising the region or receiving a knife or gunshot wound to this region can rupture the hollow organs (intestines), lacerate the spleen or liver, or tear the mesentery, which suspend the intestines in this region of the body.

SIGNS, SYMPTOMS & INDICATORS:

1. Localized tenderness.
2. Difficulty in moving.
3. Obvious entrance/exit point (as in a gunshot wound).
4. Low blood pressure.
5. Rapid pulse.
6. Shallow breathing.
7. Rapid, shallow breath (which prevents excessive movement of abdominal contents).
8. Person lies very still and is WORSE with any kind of movement.
9. Bruises on the abdomen.
10. Nausea/vomiting.
11. Ashen color to the face.
12. Distention or swelling/hardness of the abdomen (internal bleeding is present).
13. Lacerations or stab wound to the area.
14. Tire or seat belt impressions over the abdomen.
15. Anxiety.

TREATMENT:

EMERGENCY MEDICAL RESPONSE:
1. Help the person lie on their back with their knees slightly flexed and support them with a pillow or blanket beneath them.
2. Loosen their clothing. Remove it in the area of injury. Treat for Shock, page 140.
3. Inspect abdomen for wounds, bullets, a knife, or other missiles that may have entered. If an entry is found, look for exit hole(s) in the person's back.
4. Look for bruises.
5. If organs are protruding from the abdomen, see Abdominal Evisceration, page 20, for steps to protect them.
6. If the person begins to vomit, turn their head to the side to keep their airway clear of vomitus—provided there is no mechanism for spinal cord injury.

HOMEOPATHIC:
1. Follow the above procedures.
2. **Aconitum Napellus 30C**, one dose every 15 minutes. Up to six doses.
3. **Bellis Perennis 30C**, one dose every 15 minutes. Up to six doses.
4. **Arnica Montana 30C**, one dose every 15 minutes. Up to six doses.
5. **Staphysagria 30C**, for severe abdominal pain. Consult a homeopath for approval.

NOTES _____

_____

_____

_____

_____

★ABDOMINAL PAIN—ACUTE★

DEFINITION: Many times the complaint is a "stomach ache." However, it may not be something so simple or straight forward as it appears. Listed below are the other possibilities for pain in the abdomen. This complaint should always be treated seriously and not just shrugged off as being mild indigestion from eating too much food.

CAUSES:

1. Appendicitis.
2. Cholecystitis (gall bladder attack).
3. Duodenal ulcer.
4. Diverticulitis.
5. Cystitis (bladder infection).
6. Kidney infection (blood in urine).
7. Kidney stone.
8. Pelvic inflammation.
9. Pancreatitis.
10. Ectopic pregnancy.

SIGNS, SYMPTOMS & INDICATORS:

1. Assess the pain. Ask the person if pain is local or diffuse.
2. Palpate the abdomen very GENTLY with three fingers. Is it: Tender when pushed upon or released? Distended? Hard? Swollen? (All of these indicate possible internal bleeding or a more serious problem.)
3. Person is reluctant to move.
4. Person curls up, knees to chest and will lie on their side.
5. Breathing is rapid and shallow, movement makes it worse.
6. Rapid pulse.
7. Blood pressure decrease.
8. Vomiting and/or nausea.
9. Constipation.
10. Hypotension or low blood pressure.

TREATMENT:

EMERGENCY MEDICAL RESPONSE:
1. Help place the person on their side in a comfortable position.
2. Palpate the abdomen very GENTLY with three fingers. Is it: Tender when pushed upon or released? Distended? Hard? Swollen? (All of these indicate possible internal bleeding or a more serious problem.)
3. Can the person relax their abdominal wall? If not, this indicates problems.

4. No food or liquid.
5. Maintain and clear the airway. Perform CPR if necessary.
6. No medications are to be taken.
7. Bleeding? Treat for shock. (See Shock, Hypovolemic, page 141.)
8. Get a good medical history from the person as soon as possible and give it to 911 responders when they arrive. Ask for foods ingested or drugs taken.

HOMEOPATHIC:
1. Follow procedures outlined above.
2. The injured person's constitutional case must be taken after diagnosis is made. No acute homeopathic remedies are to be administered. Consult with a homeopath as soon as possible, and after 911 has been called.

NOTES _____

_____

_____

_____

_____

★ALLERGIC REACTION★
(Anaphylactic Shock)
See: Shock

DEFINITION: A person is stung by a wasp, bee, or any other insect and experiences an allergic reaction to the attack. It can also be an allergic reaction to eating a certain food, such as shrimp, drinking a particular fluid, taking a particular medicine, or inhaling a particular odor.

SIGNS, SYMPTOMS & INDICATORS:

1. Swelling of the lips, tongue, or throat.
2. Wheezing (a high-pitched sound) while exhaling (breathing out).
3. Chest tightness.
4. Coughing.
5. Difficulty breathing, shortness of breath.
6. Anxiety (because they can't breathe).
7. Abdominal cramps.
8. Skin wheals or hives may appear.
9. Respiratory failure.
10. Skin may flush, itch, and turn red.
11. Cyanosis (blue color) around lips or nail beds.
12. Vascular dilation and fainting.

TREATMENT:

EMERGENCY MEDICAL RESPONSE:
NOTE: When you know it is an allergic or anaphylactic reaction, be sure to tell the 911 operator to send ADVANCED life support if available instead of BASIC life support.

1. Protect their airway. Perform CPR if necessary.
2. Place an ice bag on the sting site.
3. Remove the stinger from the skin with a credit card (scrape it across the surface of the skin) if it is a honey bee sting.
4. The person may have an epinephrine shot or oral antihistamine with them. Ask if the person has the "Eppie" shot (EpiPen or EpiPen Jr.) with them; have them take it or their oral medication.
5. Elevate extremities but keep them lying down on their back.
6. Avoid rough handling—be gentle with the person.
7. Prevent loss of body heat. Place a blanket over and possibly under them (if they are lying on the ground).
8. No food or drink. If they drink and lose consciousness they can then vomit and create an airway blockage.

HOMEOPATHIC:
1. **Apis Mellifica 30C**, one dose every 15 minutes. Up to six doses.
2. **Carbolicum Acidum 30C**, one dose every 15 minutes. Up to six doses.

SEE: Shock, page 140.

NOTES _____

_____

_____

_____

_____

★AMPUTATION★

DEFINITION: A part of the body is cut off. (See Abrasion, Scrape on skin, Avulsion, a flap of skin, Contusion, a bruise on the skin, Laceration, a cut on the skin, and Puncture wound.)

TREATMENT:

EMERGENCY MEDICAL RESPONSE:
1. Control bleeding with direct pressure on the site with a sterile compress placed over the injury. Treat for Shock, page 140.
2. If that does not work, apply indirect pressure at the radial or femoral artery site. (See Bleeding, page 38.)
3. Elevate the extremity.
4. Prevent contamination by placing a sterile dressing over the area.
5. Remove clothing over the injury and expose it to check for further injury.
6. Immobilize that part.
7. Apply a cold pack to it.
8. If there is an amputated part, place it in a ziplock bag that has been moistened by adding a few drops of water to it, wrap the amputated part in a dry sterile dressing, and put it in the ziplock bag. Place it in a cool container—not directly on ice. Keep it COOL. Give it to 911 responders when they arrive.

HOMEOPATHIC: Consult a homeopath as soon as possible after the accident for follow-up treatment.
1. **Arnica Montana 30C**, one dose every 15 minutes. Up to six doses.
2. **Aconitum Napellus 30C**, one dose every 15 minutes, for the shock of losing a limb, 90 minutes after taking the **Arnica Montana**. Up to six doses.

AFTER SURGERY
1. **Phosphorus 30C**, one dose, to alleviate symptoms of anesthesia reactions (nausea/vomiting).
2. **Arnica Montana 30C**, one dose 30 minutes after taking **Phosphorus**. Then, one dose every 15 minutes. Up to six doses.
3. **Aconitum Napellus 30C**, one dose every 15 minutes after taking **Arnica Montana**, to get rid of surgical shock. Up to six doses.
4. **Arnica Montana 30C**, as needed if there is swelling or bruising. Consult a homeopath first.
5. **Bellis Perennis 30C**, 7 days after surgery to reattach the amputated part. Consult a homeopath first.
6. **Hypericum 30C**, one dose if experiencing nerve pain.

7. Flush with **Calendula** or **Hypericum Tincture** 1:10 (diluted 1 part Calendula or Hypericum to 10 parts water, or 1 teaspoon per quart). Once clean, use sterile dressing.

NOTES _____

_____

_____

_____

_____

★ANGINA PECTORIS★

DEFINITION: The heart is deprived of sufficient oxygen for several seconds; chest pains will then occur.

CAUSES:

An attack may be triggered by physical exertion, emotional stress, a large meal, or common anxiety.

SIGNS, SYMPTOMS & INDICATORS:

1. Pain is crushing and it takes the person's breath away.
2. They may say, "It's squeezing me," or "It's like someone's standing on my chest," or "a weight," or "an elephant."
3. Pain goes away if the person sits down and rests. It increases with resumed physical activity.
4. Pain is usually felt under the sternum/breastbone and can radiate upward to the jaw, into the arms (especially the left one), down to the middle-upper region of the abdomen (pit of stomach area), or to the back. Pain will not necessarily radiate to all of these areas; perhaps only one region.
5. Pain usually lasts 3 to 8 minutes, and rarely longer than 10 minutes. (If it lasts longer than that, suspect a heart attack. Heart attack pain usually lasts a half hour or more.)
6. Shortness of breath.
7. Nausea and/or vomiting.
8. Sweaty.

TREATMENT:

EMERGENCY MEDICAL RESPONSE:
Nitroglycerin tablets, which are usually in white pill form (about half the size of an aspirin tablet), are taken sublingually (beneath the tongue), as a spray, or on the skin as a patch. Nitro relaxes the coronary arteries within seconds and the heart again receives the necessary amount of oxygen.

SIDE EFFECT: The person may get a severe headache after taking the medication.
1. Position the person—usually sitting up or lying down with the head elevated and well supported.
2. Loosen their collar or clothing.
3. Keep them warm—but not hot.

4. Ask if they take medication. If they do, get it for them—but they must put it into their mouth. Have them SIT DOWN. They may want their nitroglycerin tablet—give it to them and have them place the pill under their tongue. Nitro dilates the arteries and muscles and the heart relaxes. Wait 2 minutes.
5. If the pain is still there, have them take a second tablet. Wait 2 more minutes.
6. If pain is still there, have them take a third tablet. Wait 2 minutes. If pain is still there after a third dose, call 911. It may mean that the coronary artery is blocked off.
7. No food or drink (other than prescribed heart medication).

HOMEOPATHIC: If the person does NOT have nitroglycerin tablets available to them, look at the remedies below. If they do have nitro tablets, have them take them as instructed above, FIRST, before using a homeopathic remedy. If the nitroglycerin tablets work, do NOT give any homeopathic remedy. Refer the person to a local homeopath for consultation after the incident.

1. **Digitalis 30C**, every 15 minutes. Up to six doses.
2. **Cactus Grandiflorus 30C**, every 15 minutes. Up to six doses.
3. **Aconitum Napellus 30C**, every 15 minutes. Up to six doses.
4. **Arnica Montana 30C**, every 15 minutes. Up to six doses.

NOTES _____

_____

_____

_____

_____

★ASTHMA★

DEFINITION: A disease of the lungs characterized by muscle spasms that occur in the small air passageways and the production of mucus that results in airway obstruction. The attack restricts or closes down the bronchioles in the lungs and slows air flow going OUT of the lungs. The problem is getting the carbon dioxide out of the lungs. Six million Americans have this disease and more and more children are becoming asthmatic each year. Four to five thousand die of this each year.

SIGNS, SYMPTOMS & INDICATORS:

1. Varying degrees of respiratory distress—depending upon severity and duration of the episode.
2. Fast, shallow breathing.
3. Audible wheezing.
4. Wants to sit up and forward.
5. Anxious.
6. May be struggling to breathe.
7. They wheeze—a high-pitched, whistling breath sound that is heard on expiration or exhalation of each breath.
8. Chest may appear inflated.
9. Uses accessory muscles of chest to breathe.
10. There is 'dry' and 'wet' asthma. In dry, little mucus is dislodged. In wet, there may be plenty of thick, stringy mucus coughed up during an attack.
11. Pulse rate may be normal or elevated.
12. Blood pressure may be slightly elevated.

TREATMENT:

EMERGENCY MEDICAL RESPONSE:

1. You may hear wheezing on exhalation of breath. This is frightening and tiring to the person.
2. Pulse rate may be normal or elevated.
3. Blood pressure may be slightly elevated.
4. Allow the person to sit up or remain in a position of comfort.
5. If oxygen is available, administer it.
6. Ask if the person carries an "Eppie" or epinephrine shot (EpiPen or EpiPen Jr.) with them (some do). If they do, have them administer it to themselves, if possible. Be warned that the effects of the "Eppie" shot will cause violent heart palpitations, shaking, and trembling— so be prepared. It will eventually ease off. NOTE: Elderly people should check with their doctor first as this may not be a recommended procedure for them.

7. If the "Eppie" shot does not stop the asthma attack, be prepared to perform CPR.
8. If they have any medication, have them take it.

HOMEOPATHIC: Try their own medication first. If it does not work, go to a homeopathic remedy. Do not place drops in mouth. Place on inside of wrist. Seek homeopathic treatment as soon after the attack as possible.

1. **Antimonium Tartaricum 30C**, every 15 minutes. Up to six doses.
2. **Arsenicum Album 30C**, every 15 minutes. Up to six doses.
3. **Apis Mellifica 30C** (if an allergy to a bite/sting/food), every 15 minutes. Up to six doses.
4. **Aconitum Napellus 30C** (for panic on the child's part), every 15 minutes. Up to six doses.

SEE: Shortness of Breath (Dyspnea), page 144.

NOTES _____

_____

_____

_____

_____

★BITES★
(Wild Animal or Human)

DEFINITION: Any kind of domestic or wild animal bite can be quite dangerous, due to the possibility of rabies, especially with raccoons, squirrels, skunks, bats, foxes, coyotes, and dogs, to name a few. However, a HUMAN bite is dangerous for many reasons: the transmission of HIV, AIDS, or Hepatitis B are examples. Plus, the human mouth is one of the dirtiest and most germ laden! The spread of infection from a human bite is very dangerous. Never treat a human bite lightly. Seek medical treatment as soon as possible.

TREATMENT for Human Bite:

EMERGENCY MEDICAL RESPONSE:
1. Stop any bleeding with direct pressure. Splint or bandage the bite location and keep it immobilized.
2. Use a dry, sterile dressing.
3. Transport to a hospital so the bite can be cleaned surgically and antibiotic therapy can be given by the doctor.

HOMEOPATHIC:
1. Go to the doctor or emergency room and allow them to do what they need to do first.
2. Then, put 1 teaspoon of **Calendula** or **Hypericum Tincture** in a quart of water (1:10) and vigorously flush the area three times daily with this application. NOTE: If the wound site is a puncture wound, do NOT use Calendula Tincture. Instead, use only Hypericum Tincture to flush the wound site.
3. **Arnica Montana 30C**, each dose an hour apart, for swelling, tissue damage, and shock. Up to six doses.
4. If the wound becomes infected, see a doctor, plus take **Pyrogenium 30C**, one dose three times daily for one day. See your MD and consult a homeopath.
5. Get tested at the appropriate times for Hepatitis B, HIV, and AIDS. Get the person who bit you tested on these three disease forms. If you test positive, see your homeopath immediately for follow-up homeopathic constitutional treatment.

TREATMENT for SMALL Wild Animal Bites:

(Includes dog bites)

EMERGENCY MEDICAL RESPONSE:

1. Stop any bleeding with a dry sterile dressing and with direct pressure over the wound site. If that does not work, apply indirect pressure on either the brachial or femoral artery. (See Bleeding, page 38.)
2. Flush the wound site with clean water for at least 3 minutes. Then wash with soap and clean water. If you have access to a turkey baster, squirt the fluid into the wound under as much pressure as possible. Bandage the bite location and keep it immobilized.
3. Splint and immobilize the area, if possible.
4. Treat for shock if necessary. (See Shock, page 140.)
5. Check their breathing. If they have stopped, perform CPR.
6. Transport to a hospital so the wound can be cleaned surgically and appropriate antibiotic therapy can be given.

LATER, with dog bites and rabies concerns:

1. Check with local authorities for specifics. If the person is bitten by any animal, there must be concern for rabies. Trap the animal or dog the best you can, without being bitten yourself. Call your city or county animal control with a description of the animal. If a dog, find out who it belongs to and get their address. Report this information to your health department officials as soon as possible.
2. Rabies, if left untreated, will kill a person.
3. Get immediate emergency medical attention.
4. Wash and flush wound as above. This will reduce possible rabies infection by 50%!
5. Any unprovoked attacks by any animal should be considered dangerous, as they may have rabies. Even if you are not bitten, report this as soon as possible to health department officials.
6. Rabies has a long incubation period, but head wounds will show the symptoms much sooner.

TREATMENT for LARGE Wild Animal Bites:

(Bear, alligator, bull, buffalo, large cat—cougar/lynx, or boar/peccary)

EMERGENCY MEDICAL RESPONSE: If you are in the woods or an area where help is not nearby.

1. Check the area for everyone's safety, especially you. If it is a GRIZZLY bear, do NOT look it in the eye and do NOT run. Just slowly back away from the person and the bear. When the bear leaves, go care for the person. If you are confronted with a BLACK or BROWN bear, cougar/lynx, make a lot of noise—yell, scream, wave your arms, and show very aggressive behavior toward it. The animal will usually leave and then you can care for the person.
2. Check their airway, breathing, and pulse. If not breathing, perform CPR.
3. Assess for multiple, major wounds. This may involve open wounds, puncture wounds, fractures, head, neck, back/spinal column, or throat injuries, or internal injuries.
4. Stop any bleeding with a dry sterile dressing and with direct pressure over the wound site. If that does not work, apply indirect pressure on either the brachial ᴏr femoral artery. (See Bleeding, page 38.)
5. Flush the wound site with clean water for at least 3 minutes. Then wash with soap and clean water. If you have access to a turkey baster, squirt the fluid into the wound under as much pressure as possible. Bandage the bite location and keep it immobilized.
6. Splint and immobilize the area, if possible.
7. Treat for shock if necessary. (See Shock, page 140.) If there are head, neck, or chest injuries, do NOT elevate the person's feet.
8. Transport to a hospital or get help as soon as the person is comfortable and you've done all you can at that time—especially if out in the woods or in some area where help is not nearby.

HOMEOPATHIC: If in the woods and not near any emergency help and assuming you are carrying a homeopathic first aid kit with you.

1. **Arnica Montana 30C**, one dose every 15 minutes for bleeding and shock. Up to six doses.
2. **Aconitum Napellus 30C**, one dose every 15 minutes if shock symptoms persist after the **Arnica Montana** has been taken six times. Up to six doses.

3. **Carbo Vegetabilis 30C,** one dose every 15 minutes if the person is having trouble breathing (along with the employment of CPR methods). Up to six doses.

NOTES _____

_____

_____

_____

_____

★BLACK WIDOW BITE★

DEFINITION: Black widows are found in all states except Alaska. Their poison is neurotoxic, which means it will affect the central nervous system. Symptoms usually subside in 48 hours. There were 63 deaths recorded from 1950 to 1960 from this spider's bite. Antivenin is used only in emergencies for the elderly or children under the age of five because it has a number of side effects.

SIGNS, SYMPTOMS & INDICATORS:

1. Injured area becomes NUMB after the bite.
2. Pain at the bite site.
3. Severe cramping—VERY painful and agonizing.
4. Board-like rigidity of the abdominal muscles.
5. Tightness in the chest.
6. Difficulty breathing—this occurs over a 24-hour period.
7. Dizziness.
8. Sweating.
9. Vomiting.
10. Nausea.
11. Skin rashes.

TREATMENT:

EMERGENCY MEDICAL RESPONSE:
1. Place ice on the bite area (place a towel between the ice bag and skin). Treat for Shock, page 140.
2. Antivenin shot (see above definition) on MD's approval.

HOMEOPATHIC: Consult a homeopath for treatment.
1. **Lachesis 30C**, one dose every 15 minutes.
2. **Latrodectus Mactans 30C**, one dose if **Lachesis** does not work—this is potentized Black Widow and acts like antivenin—without the side effects. Once every 15 minutes. Up to six doses.
3. **Ledum 30C**, one dose every 15 minutes, if bite site is COLD to the touch and the pain and swelling feels better from the application of ice. Up to six doses.

NOTES _____

_____

_____

_____

★BLEEDING★

DEFINITION: Bleeding can be a major emergency and can even be life threatening. Note that there are different types of bleeding and some are life threatening, while others can give you time to get to the emergency room or to call 911. **Bright red blood** that is spurting or pulsing out of a wound means an artery has been torn open. This type of bleeding is life threatening and must be worked with immediately. A person can lose a pint of blood in 15 to 20 minutes in such a case. If the **blood is flowing slower and is a darker red color**, that means a vein has been torn open. This is not as serious, but can be over a longer period of time. An artery that is cut at an angle will usually automatically seal itself off in a few minutes. One that receives a straight cut cannot close off and these become bleeders that require immediate attention from you in the form of direct and/or indirect pressure to stop hemorrhaging. See page 12 for an illustration of the main pressure points, the brachial or femoral artery locations.

TREATMENT:

EMERGENCY MEDICAL RESPONSE:
1. If the person is unconscious or bleeding is serious, call 911.
2. Make sure the person is breathing. If not, perform CPR.
3. Observe the wound. Locate the source of bleeding.
4. With a compress, and using the flat of your hand, place it over the wound and apply DIRECT (and continuous) pressure. If it continues to bleed, place another compress over it. Do NOT ever remove the previous compresses (blood coagulates beneath it and if you take the compress off, you rip off the clotting efforts of the body with it). If a neck wound, do not shut off breathing.
5. Elevate the arm or leg that is bleeding. If a chest injury, elevate the head (providing there is no head or neck injury).
6. If bleeding does not stop, go to one of two places known as **indirect pressure points**. One of these is the brachial artery on the upper, inside of a person's arm. Pinch between the person's biceps and triceps area on the inner side of the arm as tightly as you can with your hand and keep the pressure continuously applied to this area. See page 12 for illustration.

   The other area is the femoral artery, which is found where the leg attaches to the trunk of the body. Place the palm of your hand down, firmly, on the femoral artery (if bleeding is on the left side of the body, it would be the left femoral artery—or if on the right, use the right femoral artery). Pressure must be kept on until 911 help arrives—never loosen your pressure. If you get tired, have another person do it for you and change off until help arrives.

7. If you have a blood pressure cuff and there is bleeding from an extremity, place the cuff just above the wound and inflate it just enough to halt the bleeding. Do not deflate it—allow an MD to do this at the emergency room.

8. If all else fails, providing it is an extremity wound (arm or leg), use a tourniquet. A tourniquet is almost NEVER used and if it is put on, do NOT loosen it! That would virtually ensure the loss of any limb beyond the tourniquet. A tourniquet that is applied as a last resort can damage the tissue, muscles, and nerves if applied improperly. Here's how to apply it:

    a. Use as wide a bandage as possible with padding under it. Use a blood pressure cuff (first choice) and place just above the wound and inflate just enough to halt the bleeding. Once inflated, do NOT deflate it. Let the doctor in the emergency room do that.

    b. Never use wire, rope, or a belt—it cuts into the skin and can injure nerves, muscles, and blood supply.

    c. Do not loosen the tourniquet after it is applied.

    d. Never cover the tourniquet with a bandage—leave it in full view for the 911 responders to see.

    e. Always write "TK" on adhesive tape, with the TIME the tourniquet was placed on the person. Tape to the person's forehead.

HOMEOPATHIC: The above EMERGENCY MEDICAL RESPONSE treatment should be done first with a homeopathic remedy given secondarily. It will help slow or stop bleeding more quickly.

1. **Arnica Montana 30C**, one dose every 15 minutes. Up to six doses until bleeding slows dramatically or stops. Best for arterial bleeding where it comes out in swift spurts and is a bright, red color. If slow moving and dark colored, go to **Hamamelis Virginica**.

2. **Phosphorus 30C**, same dosage as above, if **Arnica Montana** does not help halt hemorrhaging.

3. **Hamamelis Virginica 30C**, one dose every 15 minutes. Up to six doses until bleeding slows dramatically or stops. Best for venous bleeding—slow, continuous-flow bleeding with darker colored blood.

NOTES _____

_____

_____

_____

★BLUNT INJURY★

DEFINITION: The area of contact between an object and a person's body is large enough that penetration does NOT occur. The force is transmitted through the skin into the deeper tissue and organs and can possibly rupture one of them. Auto accidents are an example of this.

SIGNS, SYMPTOMS & INDICATORS:

1. Tenderness.
2. Swelling.
3. Bruising.
4. Deformity.
5. Loss of function.

TREATMENT:

EMERGENCY MEDICAL RESPONSE:
1. **Call 911. Safety for yourself first—evaluate all possible dangers. Make sure you do not become a victim, too.**
2. Evaluate the scene—what type of injury is it? Severity is based upon the amount of kinetic energy expended upon impact.
3. Ask the person, "What happened?" and "Where do you hurt?"

HOMEOPATHIC:

IF AN AUTO ACCIDENT:
1. **Arnica Montana 30C**, one dose every 15 minutes for hemorrhage/shock/tissue damage. Up to six doses. Consult a homeopath at the first opportunity for follow-up treatment.
2. **Aconitum Napellus 30C**, one dose every 15 minutes, if shock comes back within an hour of the accident and when the last dose of **Arnica Montana** is given. This is for deeply rooted shock. Up to six doses.

OTHER LESS TRAUMATIC ACCIDENTS:
1. **Arnica Montana 30C**, one dose every 15 minutes. Up to six doses.
2. **Bellis Perennis 30C**, if swelling/bruising is not completely gone after administration of **Arnica Montana**. Consult a homeopath first.

EYE INJURY: Consult a homeopath shortly afterward for follow-up treatment.
1. **Aconitum Napellus 30C**, one dose every half hour until swelling is reduced and pain is gone. Up to six doses.
2. If **Aconitum Napellus** does not stop it completely, go to **Symphytum 30C**, one dose per hour. Up to six doses.

3. If there is blood or hemorrhaging in the eye, **Arnica Montana 30C** or **Phosphorus 30C** or **Hamamelis Virginica 30C**, to disperse the pooling of blood in the eye. One dose every 30 minutes. Up to six doses.

NOTES _____

_____

_____

_____

_____

★BROWN RECLUSE★
SPIDER BITE

DEFINITION: Try to capture the spider or keep it for identification—but do not get bitten in the process yourself. No antivenin is available. This bite may create necrosis, or dying of the flesh. This is very dangerous and there may be a need for aggressive antibiotic treatment. Treat as soon as possible. Consult a homeopath for follow-up treatment.

SIGNS, SYMPTOMS & INDICATORS:

1. Bite is not painful until several hours afterward.
2. Skin becomes red, swollen, and tender around the bite site.
3. Skin then develops a pale, mottled cyanotic (bluish) center.
4. Over the next few days, a large cap of dead skin, fat, and debris will develop over the bite site.
5. An ulcer or crater of dead tissue will form.

TREATMENT:

EMERGENCY MEDICAL RESPONSE:
1. Wash off the area of the bite with soap and water.
2. Put a cool cloth or ice (place a towel between the ice bag and the skin) over the area.
3. Call Poison Control in your state.

HOMEOPATHIC: Consult a homeopath as soon as possible.
1. **Lachesis 30C**, one dose. If symptoms return, give again. Up to three doses in first 24-hour period. If it does not completely halt symptoms, consult a homeopath.
2. **Pyrogenium 30C**, one dose if there is a red 'stripe' moving upward away from the bite area—this is sepsis or blood poisoning. Get to the emergency room quickly. If symptoms still persist, give every 15 minutes. Up to six doses. Consult a homeopath afterward for follow-up treatment.
3. **Ledum 30C**, one dose every 15 minutes, if bite site is 'cold' feeling. Up to six doses.

NOTES _____

_____

_____

_____

★BRUISE★
(Contusion)

DEFINITION: A blunt object strikes the skin and crushes the tissue underneath. There is no break in the skin. Also known as a contusion.

TREATMENT:

EMERGENCY MEDICAL RESPONSE:
1. Direct pressure on the area.
2. Elevate the extremity.
3. Put ice or a cold pack on the site. Place a cloth barrier between the ice and the skin.
4. If a bone is fractured, splint it.

HOMEOPATHIC:
1. **Arnica Montana 30C**, one dose every 15 minutes. Up to six doses unless symptoms are alleviated before that.
2. **Symphytum 30C**, once a day for 6 days, if fracture is involved. Consult a homeopath first.
3. **Arnica oil**, external application over bruised area providing there is no broken skin. Apply twice a day until the bruise is gone.

SEE: Abrasion (a scrape on the skin), page 139, Avulsion (a flap of skin), page 27, Amputation, page 27, Puncture, page 134, Laceration (a cut on the skin), page 64, and Soft Tissue Injury, page 147.

NOTES _____

_____

_____

_____

_____

★BURNS★

DEFINITION: These are serious and are probably the most painful of all injuries. There are many types of burns, as well as degrees of burn (first, second and third). Along with the burn, the person may experience shock, breathing difficulty, or even a heart attack (from lightning or electrical jolt).

SEE: Eye Injuries, page 86 or Eye Burns, page 83.

Heat or Thermal Burns

DEFINITION: A person is burned by heat from a flame or explosion, for example. This is the most common type. They may be first, second, or three degree burns.

SIGNS, SYMPTOMS & INDICATORS:

FIRST DEGREE BURN:
1. Skin turns red but does not blister.

SECOND DEGREE BURN:
1. Blisters form on the skin.

THIRD DEGREE BURN:
1. Burned area is discolored (may be charred/blackened or chalk white in appearance).
2. Clotted blood vessels may be visible under the burned skin.
3. Subcutaneous fat may be visible (it looks white).
4. There is no feeling or pain in the area of this burn (nerve endings are destroyed).
5. Skin is dry or leathery looking.

TREATMENT:

EMERGENCY MEDICAL RESPONSE:
1. Stop the burning by smothering the flames with a blanket or rolling the person to put out the flames. You can use water. Stop, drop, and roll.
2. Check to see if they are breathing. If not, proceed with CPR.
3. Remove any smoldering clothes still on them. Do NOT remove any clothing stuck to the skin. If skin is still hot, place a wet dressing on top of the area. Do not do this for more than 10 minutes. Immerse only the part that is burning, as water is a source of infection to the burned area.
4. Cover the area with a DRY gauze or a clean, dry sheet.

5. Elevate legs.
6. Do NOT use any ointments, medications, or salves. Do not remove blisters or skin from the person. Treat for Shock, page 140.

HOMEOPATHIC:

NOTE: If wrists have been burned, and the patient is unconscious, do NOT place the homeopathic dilution drop on wrist. Place drop behind the ear (if not burned) and gently rub onto the skin. If the person is conscious, give one drop in their mouth, instead.

1. **Aconitum Napellus 30C**, one dose every 15 minutes for shock and pain from injury. Up to six doses.
2. Water diluted with either **Hypericum** or **Calendula Tincture** (1 teaspoon per quart of water or 1:10 ratio)—skin must not be broken—do this for no more than 10 minutes of flushing. Afterward, place a compress across the first degree burned area.

LATER:

1. FIRST DEGREE BURN: **Cantharis 30C**, one dose four times a day for one day. Or **Urtica Urens 30C**, same dosage, if burn continues to sting. See a homeopath.
2. SECOND DEGREE BURN: **Cantharis 30C**, one dose four times a day for one day. Or **Kali Bichromicum 30C**, same dosage. See a homeopath.
3. THIRD DEGREE BURN: **Causticum 30C**, one dose four times a day for one day. Consult a homeopath for extended help on these types of burns as soon as possible.

Chemical Burns

DEFINITION: Any alkali or acid that may splash onto the body.

SIGNS, SYMPTOMS & INDICATORS:

1. Pain and possible burning sensation, depending upon the source.

TREATMENT:

EMERGENCY MEDICAL RESPONSE:

1. Flush continuously with water from a faucet—place the affected area of the body under a shower or running water for AT LEAST 15 minutes.
2. Make SURE that your own eyes are protected and do not allow any of the chemical to wash into them.
3. Stay where you are and flush, flush, flush.
4. After irrigation is complete, place a clean, dry dressing over the affected area.

HOMEOPATHIC:
NOTE: If wrists have been burned and patient is unconscious, do NOT place homeopathic dilution drop on wrist. Place drop behind the ear (if not burned) and gently rub into the skin. If person is conscious, give one drop in their mouth, instead.

1. **Causticum 30C**, one dose every 15 minutes after the above treatment has been accomplished. Up to six doses.
2. **Aconitum Napellus 30C**, one dose every 15 minutes for shock from pain. Up to six doses.
3. **Cantharis 30C**, one dose every 15 minutes. Up to six doses.

Electrical Burns

DEFINITION: This type of burn results from coming into contact with either high or low voltage electricity (such as a child playing with something metal and sticking it into an electrical outlet). Typically, there may be a small entrance point to the electrical burn, but a much larger exit point. Be sure to check opposite the entrance point. Secondly, there may be heart disruption and CPR may have to be performed. Electrical burns can cause very deep tissue damage to the muscles and you will not be aware of this. It can also cause violent muscle contractions that can fracture a bone or dislocate a joint. Compression fractures of the vertebrae are not uncommon.

SIGNS, SYMPTOMS & INDICATORS:

1. Unconsciousness.
2. Small entrance wound—large exit wound.
3. Fractures.
4. Dislocations.

TREATMENT:

EMERGENCY MEDICAL RESPONSE:
1. Call 911. Do NOT touch the person until the electricity source is off or has been removed. Call the electric company if the electrical wire is still making contact with the person. Scene safety is a must!
2. Check to make sure the person is breathing. If not, perform CPR.
3. Treat for shock. (See Shock, page 140.)

HOMEOPATHIC:
NOTE: If wrists have been burned and patient is unconscious, do NOT place homeopathic dilution drop on wrist. Place drop behind the ear (if not burned) and gently rub into the skin. If person is conscious, give one drop in their mouth, instead.

1. If unconscious but breathing, **Opium 30C**, once every 15 minutes. Up to six doses.
2. Get a professional homeopath to see the person as soon as possible after the accident.
3. If conscious but shocky, **Aconitum Napellus 30C**, once every 15 minutes. Up to six doses.

NOTES _____

_____

_____

_____

_____

★CARBON MONOXIDE★ POISONING

DEFINITION: Usually associated with cars, but also furnaces burning gas without adequate filter or ventilation, or industrial sites are the most common sources for this type of poisoning. Fumes from paint strippers contain methylene chloride which is metabolized into CO_2 by the body with severe consequences. Carbon monoxide can kill people. This is an ODORLESS gas.

SIGNS, SYMPTOMS & INDICATORS:

1. Odorless.
2. Causes no skin irritation or damage to the lungs.
3. Headache.
4. Nausea and/or vomiting.
5. Weakness.
6. All individuals in a family may complain of flu-like symptoms.
7. Cherry red skin—but this is a rare and unreliable diagnostic sign.
8. Collapse by the individual, coma, and death.

TREATMENT:

EMERGENCY MEDICAL RESPONSE:
1. Protect yourself from possible fumes first.
2. Remove the person from the contaminated area and into open air.
3. Perform CPR if necessary.

HOMEOPATHIC: Consult a homeopath after examination by an MD.
1. **Carbo Vegetabilis 30C**, one dose every 15 minutes until person stabilizes. Up to six doses.
2. **Opium 30C**, one dose every 15 minutes until person stabilizes. Up to six doses.

NOTES _____

_____

_____

_____

★CHEST INJURIES★

DEFINITION: A chest injury can be "open" (something penetrates the chest cavity, such as a knife or a bullet) or "closed" (usually caused by blunt trauma such as striking a car steering wheel, or being struck or hit by a falling object).

SIGNS, SYMPTOMS & INDICATORS:

1. Pain at the site of the injury.
2. Pain localized around the site of the injury that is aggravated or occurs when the person breathes (pleuritic pain or pleurisy).
3. Shortness of breath. Shallow breathing.
4. Failure of one or both sides of the chest to expand normally with inhalation.
5. Coughing up blood (hemoptysis).
6. Pulse is weak and rapid.
7. Blood pressure is low.
8. Cyanotic (bluish colored) around mouth or the nail beds, and possibly the face.
9. Bruising, swelling, or localized pain at the site of the injury.
10. Chest has a paradoxical motion. (See Flail Chest.)
11. Signs of shock. (See Shock, Hypovolemic, page 141 and Respiratory, page 143.)

CAUSES:

1. Loss of central nervous system control due to damage to the brain or spinal cord.
2. Obstruction in the airway.
3. Lung is compressed by either blood or air (in the pleural space).
4. Chest wall is damaged due to the sustained trauma.

TREATMENT:

1. Protect the airway. Perform CPR if necessary.
2. Control bleeding at external sites with direct pressure and sterile compress.
3. Cover penetrating chest wound with an occluded dressing. (You can use tinfoil or heavy plastic—place it over the area and tape it to the uninjured skin on all four sides. At the bottom of it, open a 2-inch area to allow for oxygen to be drawn inward and outward.)

Flail Chest Injury

See: Rib Fracture

DEFINITION: An injury in which three or more ribs are broken in two or more places. As the person breathes in, the ribs collapse against the lungs. This is known as 'paradoxical motion.'

SIGNS, SYMPTOMS & INDICATORS:

1. Chest wall does not rise properly, moving inward when inhaling— this is paradoxical motion.
2. Severe hypoxia (shortage of oxygen).
3. Cyanosis (bluish color) to the nail beds or around the mouth.
4. Pulmonary contusion (bruise to the lung) can occur directly beneath the flail segment.

TREATMENT:

EMERGENCY MEDICAL RESPONSE:
1. Stabilize the area with bulky dressings (a pillow will do) and bandage gently over that area until help arrives.

HOMEOPATHIC:
1. **Aconitum Napellus 30C**, one dose, for the shock.
2. **Arnica Montana 30C**, one dose every 15 minutes. Up to six doses if bleeding or hemorrhaging are involved, along with shock.
3. **Symphytum 30C**, to speed healing of bone up to maximum. Consult a homeopath first on this before initiating.

Pericardial Tamponade

DEFINITION: A leak from one of the vessels just above the heart, due to trauma or possibly infection. The blood leaks into the tough, fibrous pericardial sac that goes around and protects the heart. The excess blood squeezes inward on the heart, and the heart cannot pump adequate blood through the body. The person can die from a heart attack.

SIGNS, SYMPTOMS & INDICATORS:

1. Weak pulse, and it is getting weaker.
2. Jugular veins are distended and congested in upper part of body, especially in the neck region.
3. Shock—treat for Cardiogenic Shock, page 141.
4. Blood pressure—systolic and dystolic readings move toward one another—"narrowing of pulse pressure."

TREATMENT:

EMERGENCY MEDICAL RESPONSE:
1. Advanced Life Support is needed—a paramedic may need to stick a needle into the pericardial sac and draw the blood out. Only a paramedic or MD can perform this procedure.
2. Treat for cardiogenic shock. (See Shock, Cardiogenic, page 141.)

HOMEOPATHIC:
1. **Arnica Montana 30C**, one dose every 15 minutes. Up to six doses until person is stabilized.
2. **Cactus Grandiflorus 30C**, one dose every 15 minutes. Up to six doses for rupture of the blood vessels around the heart.

Pneumo-Thorax

DEFINITION: Air in the chest is OUTSIDE of the lungs. It is in the pleural space. If it is a penetrating chest wound, the air comes in from the outside. If a 'closed' injury, such as a broken rib which punctures the lung and starts leaking air into the pleural space, the same symptoms occur. Check for EQUAL breath sounds in the lungs—unequal sounds are a sign for this type of injury.

SIGNS, SYMPTOMS & INDICATORS:

SEE: Chest Injuries, page 49.

TREATMENT:

EMERGENCY MEDICAL RESPONSE:
1. Advanced Life Support is needed.

HOMEOPATHIC: See Tension Pneumo-Thorax, page 52. Consult a homeopath for ongoing treatment.

Spontaneous Pneumo-Thorax

DEFINITION: The presence of air in the chest cavity from a rupture of a congenitally weak area of the surface of the lungs. A deformity of the lung. Usually happens to boys in their late teens or twenties if they are thin and tall.

SIGNS, SYMPTOMS & INDICATORS:

1. May feel a pain or twinge in their chest—they may tell you they feel 'funny' for a while, and then they let it pass.

TREATMENT:

EMERGENCY MEDICAL RESPONSE:
1. See a doctor right away.

HOMEOPATHIC:
1. See Tension Pneumo-Thorax, page 52. Consult with a homeopath for ongoing treatment.

Tension Pneumo-Thorax

DEFINITION: Air leaks into the chest, filling up the pleural space, and compressing the lung and then the heart, arteries, and the other lung.

SIGNS, SYMPTOMS & INDICATORS:

1. Severe, progressive breathing distress.
2. Weak pulse.
3. Rapidly falling blood pressure.
4. Bulging of tissues of the chest wall between the ribs and above the collar bones.
5. Distention or swelling of the veins of the neck.
6. Cyanosis (bluish color) around mouth or nail beds.

TREATMENT:

EMERGENCY MEDICAL RESPONSE:
1. Call 911.
2. Keep the airway open. Perform CPR if necessary.
3. Keep the person as calm as possible.

HOMEOPATHIC:
1. **Stannum 30C**, one dose every 15 minutes. Up to six doses or until stabilized.
2. **Phosphorus 30C**, one dose every 15 minutes. Up to six doses.

NOTES _____

_____

_____

_____

_____

_____

_____

★CHOKING★

DEFINITION: Using the Heimlich Maneuver is essential when someone is choking. Follow the steps below.

TREATMENT:

EMERGENCY MEDICAL RESPONSE:

1. Ask the person, "Are you choking?" If they are able to speak, talk, or breathe, do NOTHING. No slapping on the back and do NOT probe their mouth with your fingers (you can push the lodged object further back into their throat this way).

2. If they cannot breathe, stand behind them, and wrap your arms around their waist. Make a fist, with the thumb side against the stomach (well below the end of the sternum and just above their belly button). Make sure it is below the sternum and never on the sternum or you'll crack it.

3. Pull your fist in a quick, UPWARD thrust into person's stomach. Do it five times in swift succession. Check to see if the obstruction has cleared the person's throat. (If the person goes unconscious, call 911). Repeat the procedure if the person is still conscious and the object is still lodged in their throat.

4. If an adult and UNCONSCIOUS (cannot be done with a child or an infant), position the person on their back and check their airway. You can open the person's mouth by grasping their tongue and lower jaw between your thumb and index finger and lifting. Quickly and gently sweep your index finger into their mouth at the base of their tongue to remove the object from their throat.

5. Using CPR, tilt their head back, lift the chin, and pinch the person's nose shut. Deliver two slow breaths into the person. If the airway is blocked and air will not go into their lungs, then …

6. Straddle the person's thighs with your legs. Put the heel of your hand well below the end of the sternum and just above the person's belly button. Place your other hand directly on top of your first hand with fingers pointed toward the person's head. Press upward with five quick, successive thrusts. Open the person's mouth and clear it of any debris you find.

7. If the person is still not breathing, tilt their head back, pinch their nose shut, and deliver two breaths of air. If the airway is still blocked, perform the stomach thrusts again. If the airway is not blocked, check for a pulse alongside the person's neck with your two fingers. If no pulse, perform CPR. If there is a pulse but person is not breathing, continue giving a breath every 5 seconds for an adult, and every 3 seconds for a child or an infant.

HOMEOPATHIC:

1. **Carbo Vegetabilis 30C**, if conscious and **after** object is removed from throat, once every 15 minutes. Up to six doses. Place a drop on the inside of the wrist or behind the ear and rub into the skin.
2. **Aconitum Napellus 30C**, one dose, if conscious and **after** the object is removed from throat, but still in shock over the incident. Place a drop on inside of the wrist or behind the ear and rub into the skin.

NOTES _____

_____

_____

_____

_____

★COMPRESSION INJURY★

DEFINITION: A 'crushing' injury where application and force occurs to the body (tissue injury) over a long period of time. Being trapped inside a car during an accident is an example of this.

SIGNS, SYMPTOMS & INDICATORS:

1. Tenderness.
2. Swelling.
3. Bruising.
4. Deformity.
5. Loss of function.

TREATMENT:

EMERGENCY MEDICAL RESPONSE:

1. Call 911. **Safety for yourself first—evaluate all possible dangers. Make sure there are none—otherwise, you become a victim, too.**
2. Evaluate the scene—what type of injury is it? Severity of the injury is based upon the kinetic energy expended upon impact.
3. Keep the person as calm as possible until 911 help arrives.
4. Ask the person, "What happened?" and "Where do you hurt?"

HOMEOPATHIC:

IF AN AUTO ACCIDENT:

1. **Arnica Montana 30C**, one dose every 15 minutes for hemorrhage/shock/tissue damage. Up to six doses.
2. **Aconitum Napellus 30C**, one dose every 15 minutes if shock comes back within one hour of the accident and last dose of **Arnica Montana**. Up to six doses. This is for deeply rooted shock. Consult a homeopath as soon as possible.
3. **Hypericum** for damage to nerves during compression. Consult a homeopath as soon as possible.

OTHER LESS TRAUMATIC ACCIDENTS:

1. **Arnica Montana 30C**, one dose every 15 minutes. Up to six doses.
2. **Bellis Perennis 30C**, if swelling/bruising is not completely gone after the administration of **Arnica Montana**. Consult a homeopath first.

NOTES _____

_____

_____

_____

★CONCUSSION★

See: Head Injury

DEFINITION: A temporary loss of some or all of the brain functions without physical damage occurring to the brain. A concussion is usually short in duration. They may see stars, or they may be unconscious and even stop breathing for a short amount of time.

TREATMENT:

EMERGENCY MEDICAL RESPONSE:
1. Do NOT move the person.
2. Make sure they are breathing. If not, perform CPR. Use modified jaw thrust. See page 18 for illustration.
3. Do not move or elevate the head or neck region.
4. Try to keep the entire body stable—do not move them! However, if you must move them, it takes two, preferably three people, to perform this maneuver known as a log roll—roll the person toward you without moving their head, neck, or back out of a straight line, as if they were a log. It takes one person to stabilize neck/head and the second and/or third person to pull at the arm/hip and then the knee/ankle area, in order to roll them over in one fluid, stable motion. See page 16 for illustration.

HOMEOPATHIC: Consult a homeopath immediately.
1. **Arnica Montana 30C**, one dose every 15 minutes. Up to six doses. If unconscious, place a drop of the dilution on inside of wrist and rub in. Later, after stabilized ...
2. **Helleborus 30C**. Consult with a homeopath first.

NOTES _____

_____

_____

_____

_____

★CONGESTIVE HEART★ FAILURE

See: Heart Attack, General

DEFINITION: Heart failure occurs when the muscles are damaged by infarction (death of tissue due to lack of oxygen) or other diseases that impede the heart's ability to pump blood throughout the body. May occur hours or days after a heart attack.

SIGNS, SYMPTOMS & INDICATORS:

1. Pulmonary edema (fluid filling the lungs). The person has frothy, pink sputum (fluid spit or coughed up from lungs).
2. Shortness of breath.
3. Localized edema (swelling) of hands and particularly the lower legs, ankle, and foot region (known as 'pedal [foot] edema').
4. Distended neck veins even if the person is sitting down.
5. The person wants to sit or stand up in order to decrease the effort to breathe. They are much worse when lying down.
6. Chest pain may or may not be present.
7. Normal to somewhat high blood pressure.
8. Breathing is rapid and shallow.
9. Stethoscope to chest: You will hear the sound of air bubbling through the fluid in the alveoli and bronchi. The sounds are called *rales*—it sounds like rattles. Or a sound like sand falling on an empty tin can. May also hear wheezing. Place stethoscope on the person's back to hear these sounds much more clearly than on the chest.

TREATMENT:

EMERGENCY MEDICAL RESPONSE:
1. Allow the person to remain in upright position with legs hanging down.
2. Calm and reassure the person.
3. Gather up any medications the person is taking and give them to the 911 responders. Give to the person if they ask for them.

HOMEOPATHIC: After the person has taken their medication and it does not work. Consult a homeopath for follow-up treatment.
1. **Cactus Grandiflorus 30C**, one dose every 15 minutes as needed until the person can reach a hospital. Up to six doses.
2. **Carbo Vegetabilis 30C**, one dose every 15 minutes, if oxygen is needed. Give as needed until help arrives. Up to six doses.

3. **Aconitum Napellus 30C**, one dose every 15 minutes for anxiety or panic. Up to six doses.
4. **Glonoine 30C**, one dose every 15 minutes. Up to six doses.

NOTES _____

_____

_____

_____

_____

★CORAL SNAKE BITE★

DEFINITION: This snake is a member of the Cobra family. It is a small, colorful (red/yellow/black bands that encircle its body) venomous reptile. It is often confused with the king snake, which has similar coloring but is not poisonous. Coral snakes have red bands bordered by yellow or white, whereas king snakes have red bands bordered by black. "Red on yellow, dangerous fellow," and "red on black, friend of Jack." The coral snake has a small mouth and usually only bites a finger or toe as a result. There may be one or more puncture sites or scratch-like wounds at the site. This poison is a neurotoxin that paralyzes the central nervous system. There is antivenin available; it is known as *Micrurus fulvius*.

SIGNS, SYMPTOMS & INDICATORS:

1. There are no or very minimal physical symptoms of the bite. Instead, bizarre behavior will occur within a few hours.
2. Progressive paralysis of eye movements and breathing.
3. Muscular incoordination.
4. Weakness and lethargy.
5. Increased salivation.
6. Difficulty swallowing.
7. Visual disturbances.
8. Fear of pain, of a stroke, of disease, of snakes, depression, wants solitude/to be left alone, fear of being left alone because something terrible might happen, angry about one's self, doesn't want to be spoken to (this is homeopathic information).

TREATMENT:

EMERGENCY MEDICAL RESPONSE:
1. Quietly reassure the person. The calmer you are, the more calm they will be in response. Treat for Shock, page 140.
2. Flush the area of bite with one to two quarts of warm, soapy water and wash away any poison left on the skin.
3. Splint extremity to minimize any movement.
4. Keep person warm and elevate lower extremities to prevent shock.
5. Keep bite site BELOW the heart level.
6. Give person nothing by mouth.
7. Call 911 and let them know it is a coral snake bite while the ambulance is en route to your home.
8. Perform CPR if necessary.

HOMEOPATHIC:
1. **Lachesis 30C**, one dose every 15 minutes. Up to six doses.
2. **Elaps Corallinus 30C**, one dose every 15 minutes. Up to six doses. This is potentized coral snake venom.
3. **Crotalus Horridus 30C**, one dose and wait 15 minutes. If bleeding from site or other orifices does not stop, continue one dose every 15 minutes. Up to six doses.

NOTES _____

_____

_____

_____

_____

★CROUP★

DEFINITION: A viral infection in infants and children that causes swelling of the lining of the larynx. It is usually characterized by a barking, brassy type of cough. This can be life threatening if the swelling partially or completely closes off the trachea and limits or stops breathing.

SIGNS, SYMPTOMS & INDICATORS:

1. Spasmodic, barking cough.
2. Hoarseness.
3. Stridor—a harsh, high-pitched sound that occurs on inhalation or inspiration of breath. A keynote symptom.
4. Fever—usually in half of the cases.
5. Usually occurs at night. Worsens at night.
6. Breathing is fast and shallow.
7. Respiratory distress.
8. Cyanosis—blueness around mouth or fingernail beds.
9. Fatigue brought on due to lack of oxygen.
10. Dehydration.

TREATMENT:

EMERGENCY MEDICAL RESPONSE:

1. Call 911 if respiration is difficult.
2. Do NOT put anything (including your fingers) into the child's mouth. It may spasm the larynx and complete airway obstruction and they cannot breathe.
3. Put the child or infant into a 'sniffing' position—head and neck are extended forward.
4. Place child on humidification—warm stream vaporizer or humidifier—or get them into a warm shower until professional help arrives. This should not go on indefinitely as the water droplets are too large and will not get rid of the mucus secretions. But in the meantime it will help stop the drying out that occurs in their upper throat region.
5. Have the child drink water or fluids and remain hydrated, if they can swallow. If not, do not force them to swallow or drink anything.
6. Rest, as fatigue and crying only aggravate the above symptoms.

HOMEOPATHIC: Seek homeopathic treatment as soon after the incident as possible.
1. **Sambucus Nigra 30C**, every 15 minutes. Up to six doses.
2. **Spongia Tosta 30C**, every 15 minutes. Up to six doses.
3. **Aconitum Napellus 30C**, for panic on the child's part, every 15 minutes. Up to six doses.

SEE: Shortness of Breath (Dyspnea).

NOTES _____

_____

_____

_____

_____

★CRUSHING INJURY★

DEFINITION: Application of force to the body tissue over a relatively long period of time. Crushing causes soft tissue damage and cuts off circulation. Auto accidents are an example of this.

SIGNS, SYMPTOMS & INDICATORS:

1. Tenderness.
2. Swelling.
3. Bruising.
4. Deformity.
5. Loss of function.

TREATMENT:

EMERGENCY MEDICAL RESPONSE:

1. Call 911. **Safety for yourself first—evaluate all possible dangers. Make sure there are none—otherwise, you become a victim, too.**
2. Evaluate the scene. What type of injury is it? Severity of the injury is based upon the kinetic energy expended upon impact.
3. Ask the person, "What happened?" and "Where do you hurt?"
4. Keep the person as calm as possible until 911 help arrives.

HOMEOPATHIC:

IF AN AUTO ACCIDENT: Consult a homeopath right away.

1. **Arnica Montana 30C**, one dose every 15 minutes for hemorrhage/ shock/tissue damage. Up to six doses. For whiplash injury, consult a homeopath first.
2. **Aconitum Napellus 30C**, one dose every 15 minutes if shock comes back within one hour of the accident and last dose of **Arnica Montana**. This is for deeply rooted shock. Up to six doses.

OTHER LESS TRAUMATIC ACCIDENTS:

1. **Arnica Montana 30C**, one dose every 15 minutes. Up to six doses.
2. **Bellis Perennis 30C**, if swelling/bruising is not completely gone after giving **Arnica Montana**. Consult a homeopath first.
3. **Ignatia Amara 30C**, one dose for hysteria after the injury.
4. **Hypericum 30C**, one dose every 15 minutes if it involves nerves and nerve-like pain. Up to six doses. Consult a homeopath if this continues after administration of this remedy.

NOTES _____

_____

_____

★CUT★
(Laceration)

See: Soft Tissue Injuries

DEFINITION: A cut produced by a sharp object such as a knife. The skin may appear smooth or jagged. It can be mild and affect only the epidermis/dermis area, or go very deep into the subcutaneous layer into the muscles, nerves, and blood supply.

SIGNS, SYMPTOMS & INDICATORS:

1. Bleeding.
2. Pain.
3. Swelling.
4. Bruising.

TREATMENT:

EMERGENCY MEDICAL RESPONSE:
1. Control bleeding—place sterile, dry dressing over wound and apply direct pressure. If that does not work, apply indirect pressure to either the brachial or femoral artery. (See Bleeding, page 38; for illustration of pressure points, see page 12.) Elevate the extremity.
2. Prevent further contamination of the injury site.
3. Immobilize the affected part.
4. Use a roller bandage to keep dressing in place. Then splint to hold in place.

HOMEOPATHIC:
1. **Tincture of Calendula** or **Hypericum**, wash and flush with 1:10 solution (1 teaspoon in a quart of water). Flush area well. This can slow the bleeding.
2. **Arnica Montana 30C**, one dose every 15 minutes for pain, swelling, and bleeding. Up to six doses.
3. For severe bleeding, **Hamamelis 30C**, one dose every 15 minutes. Up to six doses.

NOTES _____

_____

_____

_____

_____

★DEHYDRATION★

See: Heat Cramps, Heat Exhaustion, and Heat Stroke

DEFINITION: Loss of body fluids from the tissues via sweating or not drinking enough to compensate for the fluids lost. Causes for dehydration include weather conditions and extremes in temperature, diarrhea/vomiting for extended periods of time, or sweating due to exercising.

SIGNS, SYMPTOMS & INDICATORS:

MILD DEHYDRATION:
1. Fatigue and/or loss of energy.
2. Headache or body ache.
3. Thirsty.
4. Dry mouth.
5. Urine is dark colored.
6. Irritability.
7. Dizziness.

MODERATE DEHYDRATION:
1. Very dry mouth.
2. Diminished amount of urine.
3. Weakness.
4. Increased dizziness.
5. Skin is less firm.
6. Rapid and weak pulse.
7. Nausea.
8. Changes in mental state.

SEVERE/LIFE-THREATENING DEHYDRATION:
1. Loss of consciousness.
2. Sunken looking eyes.
3. Extremely dry mouth and cannot swallow.
4. Swollen tongue.
5. Delirium.

TREATMENT:

EMERGENCY MEDICAL RESPONSE—if from weather/exercise related:
1. Check breathing, pulse, and airway. If not breathing, call 911 and perform CPR. Treat for Shock, page 140.
2. Get out of the sunlight and into a shaded area.
3. If conscious, give plenty of fluids. You can use fruit juice or other commercial sports drinks such as Gatorade if available. If not, use water.

4. Do not give alcohol, caffeine drinks (colas, tea, coffee), or milk products.

EMERGENCY MEDICAL RESPONSE—if from diarrhea/vomiting:

1. Check breathing, pulse, and airway. If no pulse, perform CPR.
2. If conscious, give clear liquids in small sipping amounts. You can use fruit juice or other commercial sports drinks such as Gatorade if available. If not, use water.
3. No milk products or solid food should be given.
4. Do not stop any prescribed medications.

HOMEOPATHIC:

1. **Glonoine 30C**, one dose every 15 minutes. Up to six doses.
2. **Belladonna 30C**, one dose every 15 minutes. Up to six doses.

NOTES _____

_____

_____

_____

_____

★DIABETES★

DEFINITION: Insulin, a hormone secreted by the pancreas, is needed to break down glucose from foods we eat into sugar for energy. Diabetes limits the ability of insulin to break down glucose into usable sugar. There are two conditions a diabetic may get into: **insulin shock** or a **diabetic coma**.

Diabetic Coma

DEFINITION: There is plenty of glucose available in the body, but not enough insulin to break it down into usable sugar. This condition takes a number of days to develop.

SIGNS, SYMPTOMS & INDICATORS:

1. Fruity, acetone, or sweet odor to the breath.
2. Air hunger—they keep sighing—blowing off the acidosis/ketoses created by the condition.
3. Rapid, weak pulse.
4. Skin is dry and red.
5. Blood pressure is normal or a little below normal.
6. Level of consciousness may go from alert to unconscious to coma.
7. Slow onset of many days before a coma occurs.

TREATMENT:

EMERGENCY MEDICAL RESPONSE:
1. Give glucose gel by mouth if conscious, or let them drink orange juice.
2. Protect their airway. Perform CPR if necessary.

HOMEOPATHIC:
1. Follow the above procedures. No homeopathic remedy is to be given. See a homeopath for constitutional treatment.
2. A homeopathic case must be taken to individualize the homeopathic remedy if organic damage has not been sustained.

Insulin Shock

DEFINITION: There is plenty of insulin available in the body, but the person is not eating right or they try to go on a diet to lose weight or they exercise hard. The brain needs oxygen and sugar to survive or its cells will rapidly die off. These are typical hypoglycemic symptoms as well. Insulin shock hits hard and fast and is potentially deadly without swift action.

SIGNS, SYMPTOMS & INDICATORS:

1. Breathing is normal.
2. Blood pressure is normal.
3. Pulse is full and rapid.
4. Dizziness with a headache.
5. Skin sweaty and pale looking.
6. Level of consciousness is decreased.
7. Disoriented and/or abnormal behavior.
8. Seizure.
9. FAST onset—it is very sudden.

TREATMENT:

EMERGENCY MEDICAL RESPONSE:
1. Give glucose gel by mouth if conscious, or let them drink orange juice.
2. Protect their airway. Perform CPR if necessary.

HOMEOPATHIC:
1. Follow above procedures. No homeopathic remedy is to be given. See your homeopath for constitutional treatment after the incident.
2. A homeopathic case must be taken to individualize the homeopathic remedy toward cure if organic damage has not been sustained.

NOTES _____

_____

_____

_____

_____

★DISLOCATION★

DEFINITION: Disruption of the joint. The joint ends are no longer in contact. The most commonly dislocated joint is the shoulder.

SIGNS, SYMPTOMS & INDICATORS:

1. Deformation in the area.
2. Swelling in the joint region.
3. Pain at the joint.
4. Loss of normal joint motion or loss of use.
5. Tenderness at that joint.
6. Joint may be held in a partially flexed position—do not try to move it—splint it as is (usually a knee or shoulder joint).

TREATMENT:

EMERGENCY MEDICAL RESPONSE:

DISLOCATED SHOULDER:

1. Place a pillow between chest and affected limb.
2. Place limb in a sling.
3. Place a swathe over arm and sling to immobilize the arm.
4. Transport to the doctor.

DISLOCATED HIP:

NOTE: Usually it is the posterior (rear) hip dislocation. The person will have the hip joint flexed with their thigh rotated inward (knee pointed inward) over the midline of their body. Splint in this position—do not try to straighten this limb out.

1. Place pillows or blankets beneath the drawn-up limb.
2. Secure pillows with masking tape.

HOMEOPATHIC:

1. **Arnica Montana 30C**, one dose, BEFORE the joint is placed back in the socket by a doctor.

AFTER ADJUSTMENT:

1. **Arnica Montana 30C**, once every half hour for 3 hours, to reduce swelling at site and help muscles relax so they won't spasm.

3-6 HOURS LATER:

Consult a homeopath first before trying these suggestions:

1. **Rhus Toxicodendron 30C**, one dose, three times daily for one day—if BETTER with movement.
2. **Ruta Graveolens 30C**, one dose, three times daily for one day—if WORSE with movement.

IF THE ABOVE REMEDY DOES NOT RELIEVE SYMPTOMS:
1. **Bellis Perennis 30C**, one dose, three times daily for one day—to follow **Arnica Montana** application IF there continues to be swelling in the injured region.

IF NOTHING WORKS:
1. **Symphytum 30C**, one dose, three times daily for one day to address the ligament/capsule of the joint, directly.

NOTES _____

_____

_____

_____

_____

★DROWNING★

TREATMENT:

EMERGENCY MEDICAL RESPONSE:
1. In a cold water drowning, brain cells survive better. Perform CPR. If they vomit, turn their head to the side, clear and sweep their mouth, and continue CPR.
2. If cool and dead, perform CPR—they can have full and complete recovery without brain damage.
3. If they are warm and dead—perform CPR, but they may have brain damage.

HOMEOPATHIC: Consult a homeopath for follow-up treatment.
1. If in a coma, give **Opium 30C** or **Carbo Vegetabilis 30C**, one time. Rub on underside of wrist. Do NOT place in mouth.
2. If fluid is present in lungs after CPR and person is becoming conscious, give **Phosphorus 30C**, one dose. Rub on underside of wrist. Do NOT place in mouth.
3. If fluid is present in lungs after CPR and person is becoming conscious, give **Antimonium Tart 30C**, one dose. Rub on underside of wrist. Do NOT place in mouth.

NOTES _____

_____

_____

_____

_____

★DRUG OVERDOSE★

DEFINITION: Overdoses can occur from taking too many prescription drugs, or from an elderly person forgetting how many pills they have taken on their prescription, or from abusing 'recreational' drugs. Barbiturates, narcotics, and common prescription drugs that contain these substances are addressed separately below.

Barbiturate Poisoning/Overdose

DEFINITION: Prescription drugs containing Amabarbital, Meprobamate, Pentobarbital, Phenobarbital, and Secobarbital. More common names are Amytal, Nembutal, Seconal, and Tuinal. Marijuana, tranquilizers, inhaled solvents, and opiates such as codeine; these are known as 'downers.' Some are short acting and others are longer acting: 1–4 hours for Pentothal (thiopental) and Brevital (methohexital); 3–6 hours for Amytal (amobarbital), Seconal (secobarbital) and Nembutal (pentobarbital); 6–12 hours for Butisol (sodium butabarbital); and 12–24 hours for Luminal (phenobarbital). Barbiturates depress the central nervous system. They do not relieve pain or produce a 'high.' A typical user of barbiturates is middle aged, highly productive, and in a stressful job or home situation. Relaxation is the purpose of using such an agent.

SIGNS, SYMPTOMS & INDICATORS:

1. Respiratory depression; breathing slows.
2. Level of consciousness decreases.
3. Headache.
4. Confusion.
5. Loss of corneal reflex.
6. Delirium.
7. Drooping of eyelid or paralysis of upper eyelid.
8. Respiratory failure.
9. Coma and then death.

TREATMENT:

EMERGENCY MEDICAL RESPONSE:
1. Call 911 and perform CPR if necessary.
2. Locate pills if possible and give to 911 responders to take along to the hospital for identification.

3. Syrup of Ipecac if person is conscious to induce vomiting. If unconscious, do NOT give anything. For adults, give a 30cc dose along with two glasses of water. For children, a 15cc dose with two glasses of water. Wait 20 minutes. If the person does not vomit, repeat the same amounts.

HOMEOPATHIC: Consult a homeopath for follow-up treatment.
1. Follow the above guidelines.
2. If unconscious, use **Opium 30C**, one dose every 15 minutes. Rub one drop on inside of wrist.

Cocaine Overdose

See: Stimulant Drugs

DEFINITION: Considered an 'upper', this is one of the most abused drugs in our culture. It is known by many names: Coke, Crack, Crystal, Ice, Snow, Nose Candy, Green Gold, and Happy Trails, to name a few. It is a stimulant to the central nervous system.

SIGNS, SYMPTOMS & INDICATORS:

1. Excitement, manic behavior, cannot sit still, restless, must be in constant motion of some sort, gesticulations with hands.
2. Euphoria.
3. Talkative, non-stop babbling, loquacity.
4. Agitation, highly irritated, dangerous at times.
5. Hallucinations, think they are 10 times stronger than any other human being, think they can manage impossible feats of strength, think they can fly.
6. Cardiac arrest with overdose or continued use.
7. Death.

TREATMENT:

EMERGENCY MEDICAL RESPONSE:
1. Protect yourself, first.
2. Protect them, secondly.
3. Talk them down, keep talking.
4. Protect their airway. Perform CPR if necessary.

HOMEOPATHIC: Consult a homeopath for follow-up treatment.
1. **Tarantula Hispania 30C**, one dose every 15 minutes. Up to six doses.
2. **Nux Vomica 30C**, one dose every 15 minutes. Up to six doses.

Hallucinogenic Drugs/Overdose

DEFINITION: LSD, mescaline, peyote, Datura (jimsonweed/morning glory), and psilocybin. These induce an excitable state in the central nervous system, with either euphoric or depressive moods. LSD, in particular, has long-lasting adverse side effects such as anxiety attacks, extreme apprehensiveness, or panic states that come and go without warning (the user does not have to be on this drug to have these symptoms hit them out of nowhere). They can also get 'flashbacks' with visual illusions, sensation of distortion, or distortion of time, space, or self-image. These may last 6 to 12 months after the last ingestion of LSD. Many think they are experiencing a nervous breakdown. In serious LSD users, psychotic states or psychologic disorders may also require psychiatric care.

SIGNS, SYMPTOMS & INDICATORS:

1. Mood elevation or depression.
2. Hallucinations.
3. Dilated dyes.

TREATMENT:

EMERGENCY MEDICAL RESPONSE:
1. Protect yourself, first.
2. Protect them, secondly.
3. Talk them down, keep talking.
4. Protect their airway. Perform CPR if necessary.

HOMEOPATHIC: Consult a homeopath for follow-up treatment.
1. **Stramonium 30C**, one dose every 15 minutes. Up to six doses.
2. **Hyoscyamus 30C**, one dose every 15 minutes. Up to six doses.

Narcotic Drugs
Poisoning/Overdose

DEFINITION: Alphadropine, codeine, heroin, meperidine, methadone, morphine, opium, and propoxyphene.

SIGNS, SYMPTOMS & INDICATORS:

1. Pupils are pinpoints, tightly constricted.
2. Drowsiness.
3. Shallow respirations/breathing.
4. Uncoordinated.
5. Respiratory failure.
6. Death.

TREATMENT:

EMERGENCY MEDICAL RESPONSE:
1. Do NOT give emetics or Syrup of Ipecac.
2. Perform CPR if necessary.
3. Locate pills if possible and give to 911 responders to take along to the hospital for identification.

HOMEOPATHIC: Consult a homeopath for follow-up treatment.
1. Follow the above guidelines.
2. If unconscious, use **Opium 30C**, one dose on the way to a hospital. Rub one drop on the inner side of the wrist. After they regain consciousness:
3. **Lachesis 30C**, one dose every 15 minutes. Up to six doses.
4. **Nux Vomica 30C**, one dose every 15 minutes. Up to six doses.

Stimulant Drugs/Overdose

DEFINITION: Includes amphetamines, which are taken by truck drivers, students, and others to produce general mood elevation, suppress appetite, and prevent sleepiness. Nasal decongestants are mildly stimulating. So is caffeine, which is found in coffee, soda pop, and tea. Anti-asthmatic drugs as well as vaso-constrictors also fall into this category.

TREATMENT:

EMERGENCY MEDICAL RESPONSE:
1. Protect yourself, first.
2. Protect them, secondly.
3. Talk them down, keep talking.
4. Protect their airway. Perform CPR if necessary.

HOMEOPATHIC: Consult a homeopath for follow-up treatment.
1. **Tarantula Hispania 30C**, one dose every 15 minutes. Up to six doses.
2. **Nux Vomica 30C**, one dose every 15 minutes. Up to six doses.

NOTES _____

_____

_____

_____

_____

★EMPHYSEMA★

DEFINITION: A disease of the lungs causing dilation and destruction of the alveoli with poor exchange of oxygen and carbon dioxide.

SIGNS, SYMPTOMS & INDICATORS:

1. The person will be leaning forward; they are usually emaciated looking. They will 'tripod' or lean forward with their hands or elbows resting on their thighs to get more air into their lungs; the gravity helps them breathe better.
2. They are usually barrel chested.
3. There may be cyanosis (blueness) around their lips and nail beds of their fingers/toes.
4. They are usually wearing a nasal cannula and are on oxygen.
5. The person is in respiratory distress and they are breathing beyond the normal 12 to 20 breaths per minute.
6. Their blood pressure is slightly elevated.
7. They are tense, anxious, and panicky.
8. They will refuse to lie down because they feel like they are going to drown in the fluid of their own lungs. As a consequence, sleep deprivation.
9. They will always be sitting up in a reclining chair or semi-erect to breathe better.

TREATMENT:

EMERGENCY MEDICAL RESPONSE:
1. Reassure them, talk quietly and calmly to them. Try to help them relax.
2. If not breathing, perform CPR.
3. If the person has prescription drugs to take, help them—put the pills in their hand.
4. Place them in a position of comfort—usually they want to be in a semi-reclining or sitting up position. Do NOT lay them down.

HOMEOPATHIC: Seek homeopathic treatment as soon after the incident as possible.
1. **Carbo Vegetabilis 30C**, every 15 minutes. Up to six doses.
2. **Antimonium Tartaricum 30C**, every 15 minutes. Up to six doses.

3. **Arsenicum Album 30C**, every 15 minutes. Up to six doses.
4. **Aconitum Napellus 30C** for panic/anxiety, every 15 minutes. Up to six doses.

SEE: Shortness of Breath (Dyspnea).

NOTES _____

_____

_____

_____

_____

★EPIGLOTTITIS★

DEFINITION: A bacterial infection, usually in children, that causes swelling of the flap of tissue that protects the opening to the larynx. A severe, swift onset and a life-threatening acute illness of the greatest magnitude. Call 911 right away. Ask for an ADVANCED life support team, if available. SPEED IS VITAL!

SIGNS, SYMPTOMS & INDICATORS:

1. They will complain of a sore throat. If this flap (the epiglottis) goes into spasm, it shuts down and the child can't breathe at all.
2. Drooling and sitting forward with their neck hyper-extended. Also called the "sniffing position."
3. Drooling because it is too PAINFUL for them to swallow—this is a life-threatening condition.
4. Do NOT give liquids or food or stick anything into their mouth or throat (including your fingers).
5. Shortness of breath.
6. Fast breathing.
7. Stridor—a harsh, high-pitched sound that occurs on inhalation or inspiration of breath.
8. Restless, anxious, and distressed.
9. Starts with a sore throat, hoarseness, and frequently a fever with a very swift onset. Startlingly fast in a child who perhaps an hour earlier was healthy and fine.

TREATMENT:

EMERGENCY MEDICAL RESPONSE:

1. Call 911. Waste no time. Ask for an ADVANCED life support team if available.
2. Let the child sit forward and drool. It is too painful for them to swallow.
3. Do NOT put a tongue depressor or fingers or anything into the child's mouth. If you do, it could spasm shut the epiglottis and breathing is shut off. (If the child does go unconscious because of this, initiate normal CPR procedures.)
4. Remain calm and supportive of the child. Do not frighten the child or show your worry or anxiety for them.

HOMEOPATHIC: Rub the homeopathic dilution on the child's inner wrist—NEVER place pellets or the dilution into their mouth!!!! Use a homeopathic dilution for safety reasons. If you have none, rub Rescue Remedy on the inside of the child's wrist, instead, every 5 minutes until 911 help arrives. Seek homeopathic treatment as soon after the incident as possible.

1. **Aconitum Napellus 30C**, one dose by rubbing on inner wrist or behind the ear, once every 5 minutes for panic and anxiety. Up to six doses.
2. **Allium Cepa 30C**, one dose every 5 minutes by rubbing on inner wrist or behind the ear until help arrives. Up to six doses.
3. **Formica Rufa 30C**, one dose every 5 minutes by rubbing on inner wrist or behind the ear until help arrives. Up to six times.

SEE: Shortness of Breath (Dyspnea).

NOTES _____

_____

_____

_____

_____

★EPILEPSY★

DEFINITION: A seizure caused by an abnormal focus or activity within the brain, producing severe motor (tonic/clonic) responses or changes in consciousness. Classified as general and partial seizures—commonly known as grand mal and petite mal seizures. Classifications include nonclusive seizure (petit mal), simple partial seizure, generalized seizure (grand mal), and complex partial seizure (psychomotor seizure).

CAUSES:

1. Stroke.
2. Heart attack.
3. Head injury.
4. Drug or alcohol induced.

SIGNS, SYMPTOMS & INDICATORS:

1. Aura—the epileptic knows by feeling this, that a seizure is imminent—it can be a sound, a twitch, a feeling of dizziness, or anxiety or perception of an unusual odor that precedes the convulsions.
2. Tonic (rigid) muscular contractions that cause odd posturing of the body—they may last several minutes.
3. Clonic (repetitive) muscular activity, or spasms, may be superimposed on the tonic contractions.
4. Convulsions; jaw muscles contract (may occasionally cause epileptic to bite tongue or lips).
5. Loss of bowel or bladder control.
6. May or may not have loss of consciousness, depending upon the type of seizure experienced: grand mal—loss of consciousness; petite mal—no loss of consciousness.
7. Postictal phase—a period of exhaustion after the seizure. This phase may last 10 to 30 minutes and the person's level of consciousness is depressed. Allow them to rest.

TREATMENT:

EMERGENCY MEDICAL RESPONSE:
1. Protect the person from hurting themselves—move chairs or tables so they do not injure themselves while in a seizure.
2. Do not restrain them.
3. Do not force anything into their mouth.
4. After the seizure, roll them onto their side.
5. Get rid of bystanders—give them privacy—especially if bowel or urinary control is lost—it is highly embarrassing to the epileptic.

HOMEOPATHIC:

1. Follow the above procedures first. Do not administer any homeopathic remedy.
2. Constitutional treatment is recommended, but only after the seizure, and the person is stable. Do not give any acute homeopathic remedy.
3. Rescue Remedy is recommended, one drop rubbed on the inside of the wrist every 5 minutes until person is no longer shaken by the experience.

Generalized Seizure

DEFINITION: A grand mal seizure with all of the above symptoms, plus they lose complete consciousness.

Nonconvulsive Seizure

DEFINITION: A seizure without convulsions. The person may go into a sudden 'stare'; there is a short (seconds) lack of attention and a prompt return to full awareness. This is common in children. There is no emergency care for this, but if a teacher or parent sees this repeated behavior in a child, the child will need medical evaluation. It may be misdiagnosed as daydreaming and inattention. The outcome will be poor learning if it is not diagnosed and recognized. Homeopathic constitutional treatment should be pursued as soon as a diagnosis is made.

Simple Partial Seizure

DEFINITION: The person is awake and alert, but experiences an involuntary jerking which progresses to involve one entire side of the body or one limb. There is no emergency care indicated for this unless it progresses into a generalized seizure. It may be misdiagnosed as odd mental behavior. Constitutional homeopathic treatment should be pursued as soon as this is diagnosed.

Complex Partial Seizure

DEFINITION: The person is confused, shows random repetitive actions, may 'start' or 'stare', and is generally unresponsive with altered consciousness. This usually lasts 2 to 5 minutes. There is no memory of the seizure and there is a long post-seizure period. No emergency care is indicated for this. Just reassure the person and protect them. Do not restrain, startle, or command. Suggest gently and guide. This condition may be misdiagnosed as drug or alcohol induced behavior or a mental disease. Constitutional homeopathic treatment should be pursued as soon as this is diagnosed.

NOTES _____

_____

_____

_____

_____

★EYE BURNS★

Chemical Burns to the Eye

DEFINITION: An alkali or acid has splashed into the eye.

SIGNS, SYMPTOMS & INDICATORS:

1. Pain and possible burning sensation, depending upon the source.

TREATMENT:

EMERGENCY MEDICAL RESPONSE:
1. Flush continuously with water from a faucet—put head under faucet for AT LEAST 15 minutes. If you have saline solution it can be hooked up to a nasal cannula if both eyes are affected. Have the person lie down and place the cannula over the bridge of their nose and flush for 15 minutes with water or saline solution. You may have to gently force open the eyelids for the irrigation to be effective.
2. Make SURE that the unaffected eye does not get any of the chemical washing into it—always flush from the inner corner of the eye, outward.
3. Stay where you are and flush, flush, flush.
4. After irrigation is complete, place a clean, dry dressing over the eye and transport to the hospital.

HOMEOPATHIC: Consult a homeopath.
1. **Causticum 30C**, one dose every 15 minutes after the above treatment has been accomplished. Up to six doses.
2. **Aconitum Napellus 30C**, one dose every 15 minutes for shock from pain to the eye following **Causticum** treatment. Up to six doses.
3. **Cantharis 30C**, one dose every 15 minutes. Up to six doses.

Corneal Burns to the Eye

DEFINITION: A burn to the transparent tissue layer in front of the pupil and iris.

SIGNS, SYMPTOMS & INDICATORS:

1. Severe conjunctivitis—redness.
2. Pain begins 3 to 5 hours after exposure to source.
3. Swelling.
4. Excessive tears running from eyes.

TREATMENT:

EMERGENCY MEDICAL RESPONSE:
1. Call your physician right away for instructions. If no physician is available, go to the emergency room or call 911.

HOMEOPATHIC:
1. **Apis Mellifica 30C**, one dose as needed to control pain and swelling. Up to six doses.
2. **Causticum 30C**, one dose. Consult with homeopath first.
3. If **Apis Mellifica 30C**, one dose every hour, does not work, go to **Symphytum 30C**, one dose as needed to control pain and swelling. Up to six doses.
4. **Cantharis 30C**, one dose. Consult a homeopath first.

Light Burns to the Eye

DEFINITION: A person can receive this type of burn by looking at an eclipse (infrared burn); working with a laser, working around welding equipment, or being exposed to bright sunlight on snow or a sun lamp (all ultraviolet burns); or looking into direct sunlight for an extended period of time.

SIGNS, SYMPTOMS & INDICATORS:

1. Painless for infrared injury.
2. Painless the first 3 to 5 hours for ultraviolet exposure, but then eyes become highly painful as cornea responds to the burn.
3. Severe conjunctivitis with redness and swelling.
4. Excessive tear production.

TREATMENT:

EMERGENCY MEDICAL RESPONSE:
1. Cover each eye with a sterile, moist pad and an eye shield or cup.
2. Have the person lie down for transport to a hospital.
3. Protect the person from further exposure to bright lights of any kind.
4. The person should be examined as soon as possible by a doctor.

HOMEOPATHIC: Consult a homeopath.
1. **Apis Mellifica 30C**, one dose every 15 minutes as needed to control pain and swelling. Up to six doses.
2. **Causticum 30C**. Consult a homeopath.

3. If **Apis Mellifica 30C** does not work, go to **Symphytum 30C**, one dose every 15 minutes as needed to control pain and swelling. Up to six doses.
4. **Cantharis 30C**. Consult a homeopath.
5. **Arsenicum Album 30C**, one dose every 15 minutes for burning in the eyes due to exposure to sun, snow, or heat. Up to six doses.

Thermal Burns to the Eye

DEFINITION: The eye sustains an injury, usually from a 'flash fire' situation.

TREATMENT:

EMERGENCY MEDICAL RESPONSE:
1. Place sterile, moistened dressings (with saline solution if possible—if not, dampen with some sterile water or as a last resort, tap water) over both eyes and transport without further examination to the hospital.

HOMEOPATHIC:
1. **Aconitum Napellus 30C**, one dose every 15 minutes, for shock and pain from the injury. Up to six doses.

LATER: Consult with a homeopath first.
1. **Causticum 30C**.
2. **Cantharis 30C**.

NOTES _____

_____

_____

_____

_____

★EYE INJURIES★
See: Eye Burns

Blowout Fracture

DEFINITION: Bones around the eye are fractured.

SIGNS, SYMPTOMS & INDICATORS:

1. Double vision.
2. Pain.
3. Decreased vision.

TREATMENT:

EMERGENCY MEDICAL RESPONSE:
1. Protect eye from further injury with a metal shield or cup.
2. Cover the uninjured eye to minimize movement to the injured eye.

HOMEOPATHIC:
1. **Arnica Montana 30C**, one dose before and after surgery. Consult a homeopath for long-term follow-up treatment. May need it three times a day for 2 days after surgery. Four days later, **Bellis Perennis 30C**, three doses a day. Up to six doses.
2. **Symphytum 30C**, one time daily for 6 days to help bones mend quickly. This can be given shortly after the person comes out of surgery.

Blunt Trauma to the Eye

DEFINITION: Blunt trauma (it does not break the skin) to the eye from an outside source, such as a fist, baseball, or running into something that causes trauma to the eyeball. It can be a black eye or something more serious, such as hyphema (bleeding in the anterior chamber of the eye that may or may not obscure the iris), retinal detachment, or a blowout fracture, where the bones around the eye shatter and some of the fragments are entrapped by the muscles and hinder eye movement and motion.

SIGNS, SYMPTOMS & INDICATORS:

1. Pain.
2. Swelling.
3. Redness to the conjunctiva (the mucous membrane lining the inside of the eyelids as well as the front of the eye).

4. Bruising around the orbit of the eye (black eye).
5. Cornea may lose its smooth, wet appearance, indicating damage to this portion of the eye.

EMERGENCY MEDICAL RESPONSE—For a Black Eye:
1. Ice or cool pack GENTLY placed upon the area.

HOMEOPATHIC:
1. **Arnica Montana 30C**, one dose every hour. Up to six doses for a black eye.
2. **Aconitum Napellus 30C**, one dose every hour, is considered the "Arnica for the eye." Up to six doses.
3. **Symphytum 30C**, one dose every 15 minutes. Up to six doses for trauma to the eye. Consult a homeopath if any symptoms are still present after this time period.
4. **Hamamelis Virginica 30C**, one dose every 15 minutes. Up to six doses.

Eye Laceration or Penetration

DEFINITION: The eyelid is lacerated or cut. There may be a penetrating injury to the globe of the eye itself that you may or may not be able to see or judge.

SIGNS, SYMPTOMS & INDICATORS:

1. Bleeding from a lacerated eyelid may be profuse. If only the eyelid is injured:

EMERGENCY MEDICAL RESPONSE—For a Lacerated Eyelid:
1. Use dry sterile compress and apply gently to the injury.

HOMEOPATHIC:
1. **Arnica Montana 30C** every 15 minutes until bleeding stops. Up to six doses.

EMERGENCY MEDICAL RESPONSE—For a Penetrating Injury to the Eye:
1. Never exert pressure or manipulate the eye in any way.
2. If part of the eyeball is exposed, gently apply a moist, sterile dressing to prevent it from drying out.
3. Cover the injured eye with a protective metal shield or cup.
4. Cover the opposite eye with a bandage to decrease movement in the injured eye.

HOMEOPATHIC:

1. **Arnica Montana 30C**, one dose, before and after doctor has dislodged impaled object. Consult a homeopath for long-term follow-up treatment.
2. **Symphytum 30C**, one dose per hour afterward. Up to six doses.

Hyphema

DEFINITION: Bleeding into the anterior chamber (frontal portion of the eyeball), obscuring the iris. Blunt trauma usually creates this condition. This can indicate further damage to the eye; a doctor should be seen as soon as possible.

SIGNS, SYMPTOMS & INDICATORS:

1. Redness to the entire eye.
2. Iris may be obscured or opaque looking.

TREATMENT:

EMERGENCY MEDICAL RESPONSE:

1. Transport to a doctor for treatment or have 911 transport them.
2. Do NOT pack eye with ice—no pressure should be placed upon the injured eye.
3. If you have an eye cup, place it gently over the injured eye so that it rests on the bones around the eye. Then wrap both eyes with gauze. NOTE: Both eyes need to be wrapped or the one that is not continues to move—and so will the injured one. It is important that the injured eye not move or be stimulated.
4. Do not give aspirin or its equivalent—aspirin can cause even more bleeding into the injured eye and increased the volume of fluid within it.
5. Sometimes emergency rooms are overloaded, the staff is working double-time, and the resident on duty is not an ophthalmologist. This is where you come in and ask questions before anyone (nurse, nursing assistant, or even the resident doctor) decides to put eye drops into your child's injured eye to help examine it more closely. If the doctor in the ER is NOT an ophthalmologist, ask questions— plenty of them. If they diagnose your child as having a Hyphema, ask immediately that an ophthalmologist be contacted to back up this resident on your child's case—and be on the phone ahead of time before that resident does anything to your child. Why?

Even well-meaning residents do not remember everything about physiology and anatomy in an ER. Be extremely watchful if the RN or doctor wants to put harmless-looking eye drops in an injured person's eye. Stop them and ask what it is and why does the doctor want it done. Miotics or mydractics are CONTRA-INDICATED in a Hyphema injury. That means that ANY eye drop that is designed to dilate the pupil can NOT be used!! Miotics, such as pilocarpine and eserine, are designed to force the pupil of the eye to dilate. Mydractics, which also dilate the pupil, come from atropine, cocaine, ephedrine, euphthalmine, and homatropine.

Stop them. Ask what was ordered by the doctor. Ask if the substance that is being used is only to dilate the pupil. If it is—refuse to allow it to be done to your child or the injured party. Get the ophthalmologist to take over the case right away.

HOMEOPATHIC:

NOTE: Due to the seriousness of this condition, contact a homeopath shortly after calling 911. The potency prescribed for this condition, if wrong, can possibly cause an aggravation and an increase in fluid volume in the eye—this is not what you want. If possible, contact an opthalmologist/homeopath. See the National Center for Homeopathy directory, Appendix B, to see if there is one in your vicinity. If not, contact a homeopath and in this case, a low potency such as 6X or 6C is highly recommended—no high potencies such as a 30C, 200C, or 1M.

1. **Aconitum Napellus 30C**, one dose after the injury and before arrival at the hospital.
2. **Ledum**. Consult a homeopath first.
3. **Phosphorus**. Consult a homeopath first.
4. **Hamamelis virginica**. Consult a homeopath first.
5. **Bellis Perennis**. Consult a homeopath first.
6. **Belladonna**. Consult a homeopath first.

Retinal Detachment

DEFINITION: Separation of the inner sensory layer from the outer layer. Usually caused by a hole or break between the two layers. Can cause blindness.

SIGNS, SYMPTOMS & INDICATORS:

1. Painless.
2. Flashing lights or 'floaters' across vision.
3. Vision may be clouded or shaded.

TREATMENT:

EMERGENCY MEDICAL RESPONSE:

1. Transport to the doctor who will determine what can be done.

HOMEOPATHIC:

1. **Phosphorus 30C**, one dose every 15 minutes. Up to three doses to stop bleeding and stabilize the eye. See a homeopath for constitutional treatment shortly afterward.

NOTES   _____

_____

_____

_____

_____

★FAINTING★
(Psychogenic Shock)

DEFINITION: The only type of shock that is NOT life threatening. The blood vessels dilate and the person falls down. Once lying on their back, the blood flows back to the head and they revive on their own.

TREATMENT:

EMERGENCY MEDICAL RESPONSE:
1. Secure the airway. Perform CPR if necessary.
2. Control the bleeding—direct pressure on the wound or on indirect pressure points, radial/femoral artery, or as a last resort, a tourniquet. (See Bleeding, page 38.)
3. Elevate extremities but keep them lying down on their back.
4. Splint fractures. Pain of a broken limb can keep them in shock or deepen their shock. Splinting relieves a lot of pain, therefore reducing shock.
5. Avoid rough handling—be gentle with the person.
6. Prevent loss of body heat. Place a blanket over and possibly under them (if they are lying on the ground).
7. No food or drink. If they drink, they can lose consciousness and then vomit and create airway blockage.

HOMEOPATHIC:
1. **Ignatia Amara 30C**, one dose every 15 minutes, for hysteria, grief, loss, or anticipating treatment at ER/hospital/surgery/dentist. Up to six doses.
2. **Aconitum Napellus 30C**, one dose every 15 minutes, for those who faint at the sight of blood, or seeing a traumatic event, or due to anxiety/panic attack, or due to severe pain. Up to six doses.
3. **Arnica Montana 30C**, one dose every 15 minutes for those who faint at the slightest amount of pain. Up to six doses.
4. **Moschus 30C**, one dose every 15 minutes for hysterical fainting. Up to six doses.
5. **Nux Moschata 30C**, one dose every 15 minutes for fainting due to pain or the sight of blood. Up to six doses.

SEE: Shock, page 140.

NOTES _____

_____

_____

_____

★FOOD POISONING★

DEFINITION: There are actually THREE types of food poisoning but they get whitewashed under one label. The bacteria themselves cause the symptoms (Salmonella and Clostridium). The other type (botulism) occurs when the bacteria have produced toxins (poison).

Botulism

DEFINITION: This is the most severe variety of food poisoning. The spores of the Clostridium bacteria have grown inside contaminated food. This is food that is either not kept at a low enough temperature or not cooked at a high enough temperature. Food left out to warm up on a kitchen counter for too long can also be the cause. This form of food poisoning can kill; it attacks our neurological (nervous) system.

SIGNS, SYMPTOMS & INDICATORS:

Symptoms may not appear for upwards of 24 hours after ingestion of the contaminated food source.
1. Blurred vision.
2. Weakness.
3. Difficulty speaking.
4. Difficulty breathing.

TREATMENT:

EMERGENCY MEDICAL RESPONSE:
1. Perform CPR if necessary. Treat for Shock, page 140.

HOMEOPATHIC: Consult a homeopath immediately after going to the emergency room for medical help.
1. **Arsenicum Album 30C**, one dose every 15 minutes. Up to six doses.
2. **Carbolicum Acidum 30C**, one dose every 15 minutes. Up to six doses.
3. **Nux Vomica 30C**, one dose every 15 minutes. Up to six doses.

Ptomaine Poisoning

DEFINITION: This type of food poisoning is the direct result of the bacteria, known as Salmonella. It is also called Salmonellosis. This type of food poisoning can be eliminated with proper cleanliness procedures and proper cooking of the food at the right temperature. Some people are carriers of Salmonella and although they may not be ill from it, they can pass the Salmonella onto others through anything they touch, especially if they work in the food industry and do not use mandatory protective gloves and coverings as outlined by health department rules.

SIGNS, SYMPTOMS & INDICATORS:

Symptoms may not occur for upwards of 72 hours after ingestion.

1. Nausea.
2. Vomiting.
3. Diarrhea.
4. Fever.
5. Weakness.

TREATMENT:

EMERGENCY MEDICAL RESPONSE:
1. Perform CPR if necessary. Treat for Shock, page 140.

HOMEOPATHIC: Consult a homeopath immediately after going to the emergency room for medical help.

1. **Arsenicum Album 30C**, every 15 minutes. Up to six doses.
2. **Nux Vomica 30C**, every 15 minutes. Up to six doses.

Staphylococcus

DEFINITION: This type of food poisoning is usually seen at large functions, such as a social gathering or a church picnic event. The bacteria has had time to create toxins due to warm conditions and the food being left out too long and not refrigerated properly. Mayonnaise left at room temperature very commonly carries the staphylococcal toxins.

SIGNS, SYMPTOMS & INDICATORS:

Symptoms usually appear 1 to 3 hours after ingesting the tainted food source. It is usually over within 6 to 8 hours.

1. Nausea.
2. Vomiting.
3. Diarrhea.

TREATMENT:

EMERGENCY MEDICAL RESPONSE:
1. Perform CPR if necessary. Treat for Shock, page 140.

HOMEOPATHIC: Consult a homeopath immediately after going to the emergency room for medical help.

1. **Arsenicum Album 30C**, every 15 minutes. Up to six doses.
2. **Nux Vomica 30C**, every 15 minutes. Up to six doses.

NOTES _____

_____

_____

★FRACTURE★

See: Hip Fracture

DEFINITION: Any break or loss of continuity in a bone.

TYPES OF FRACTURE:

1. **Greenstick**—partial break of a bone; usually found in children.
2. **Transverse**—bone is broken horizontally—straight across.
3. **Oblique**—bone breaks at an angle.
4. **Comminuted**—bone is crushed.
5. **Impacted**—downward pressure on bone has jammed bones together and cracked/crushed them.
6. **Spiral**—twisted bones—seen more in sports-related injuries.

TWO VARIETIES OF FRACTURE:

1. **Open fracture**—the skin is broken. Also known as a 'compound' fracture.
2. **Closed fracture**—the skin is not broken. Also known as a 'simple' fracture.

SIGNS, SYMPTOMS & INDICATORS:

1. Deformity at the site.
2. Tenderness in the area of the break—you can press GENTLY with an index finger to find out.
3. Crepitus—grinding of broken bones with movement.
4. Discoloration—bruising.
5. Loss of use of that limb.
6. Bone fragments are exposed.

TREATMENT:

EMERGENCY MEDICAL RESPONSE:

1. If a bone is broken between joints, splint above and below the joint . Treat for Shock, page 140.
2. If a joint is fractured, splint above and below it.
3. If a mid-femur fracture, EMT or paramedics may use a traction splint after they arrive.
4. Remove all clothing to check for further fractures.
5. Cover all wounds with dressings.
6. Do NOT replace protruding bone(s).

7. If no 911 help is nearby, use a pillow around the fracture as a splint, tape it, and pad the splint(s) with a blanket or other material to fill in the voids, particularly if you use wood for splint material. If a leg is involved, splint the broken leg to the good leg. Place a blanket or material between the legs to stabilize, then tape them together.
8. Try to splint before you transport.
9. When in doubt, splint.

HOMEOPATHIC: Consult a homeopath for follow-up treatment.

1. Give **Arnica Montana 30C**, one dose every 15 minutes until shock is stabilized and for muscle/tissue damage/bleeding/shock symptoms. If no 911 help is nearby, continue to give once an hour if they are shocky. Up to eight doses or until you can reach a medical facility. If that does not stabilize their shock, go to **Aconitum Napellus 30C**, one dose every 15 minutes until shock is stabilized and for muscle/tissue damage/bleeding/shock symptoms. If no 911 help is nearby, continue to give once an hour if they are shocky. Up to eight doses or until you can reach a medical facility.
2. **Arnica Montana 30C**, for swelling and bruising afterward. Consult a homeopath first.
3. **Symphytum 30C**, restores bone growth and knitting at optimum speed. Consult a homeopath first.
4. **Calcarea Phosphorica 30C**, if healing of fractures is delayed. Consult a homeopath first.
5. One week afterward: **Bellis Perennis 30C**. Consult a homeopath first.

NOTES _____

_____

_____

_____

_____

★FROSTBITE★
(Superficial)

See: Frostnip, Frostbite (Deep), and Hypothermia

DEFINITION: The skin is frozen.

SIGNS, SYMPTOMS & INDICATORS:

1. Skin may be white, yellow, or bluish white and looks waxy.
2. Frostbitten surface is hard when touched or palpated.
3. Skin is cold feeling.

TREATMENT:

EMERGENCY MEDICAL RESPONSE:
1. Remove person from exposure.
2. Protect the frozen part—do not rub it.
3. Remove any wet or restrictive clothing.
4. Remove any rings from fingers or other jewelry.
5. Put dry, sterile dressing on the area.
6. Elevate feet. (See Shock, page 140.)

HOMEOPATHIC:
1. Follow the above procedures and …
2. **Agaricus Muscarius 30C**, one dose every 15 minutes. Up to six doses.
3. **Apis Mellifica 30C**, one dose every 15 minutes, for severe, burning pain as the skin begins to thaw. Up to six doses.
4. **Petroleum 30C**, one dose every 15 minutes. Up to six doses.

NOTES _____

_____

_____

_____

★FROSTBITE★
(Deep)

See: Frostnip, Frostbite (Superficial), and Hypothermia

DEFINITION: Not only the skin is frozen, but the tissue beneath it too.

SIGNS, SYMPTOMS & INDICATORS:

1. Skin is cold.
2. The skin, when palpated, is hard and frozen.
3. Skin may be white, yellow, or bluish white in color.
4. Blisters.
5. Area is swollen and hard.
6. Numbness to the area.
7. When returning to normal, skin will become red, purple, and blotchy looking; it is swollen and very painful.

TREATMENT:

EMERGENCY MEDICAL RESPONSE:
1. Protect the limb and do not bump it accidentally.
2. Do not break the blisters.
3. Put dry, sterile dressings across the affected surface.
4. Do not rub the area. Treat for Shock, page 140.
5. Do not try to warm up the area beyond 100° F in warm water.
6. Call 911 and ask what else you can do until help arrives. They may have further instructions for you.
7. If unconscious, protect their airway. Perform CPR if necessary.

HOMEOPATHIC: Consult a homeopath for follow-up treatment.
1. Follow the above procedures and …
2. **Agaricus Muscarius 30C**, one dose every 15 minutes. Up to six doses.
3. **Apis Mellifica 30C**, one dose every 15 minutes, for severe, burning pain as the skin begins to thaw. Up to six doses.
4. **Lachesis 30C**, one dose every hour if skin turns purple-red blotchy color. Up to six doses.
5. **Laurocerasus 30C**, one dose every 15 minutes. Up to six doses.

NOTES _____

_____

_____

_____

★FROSTNIP★

See: Frostbite (Superficial), Frostbite (Deep), and Hypothermia

DEFINITION: The skin surface is frozen but not the deeper tissue.

SIGNS, SYMPTOMS & INDICATORS:

1. Skin is blanched, waxy, or pale looking.
2. Skin is cool or cold to the touch.
3. Peeling or blistering may occur in these areas 24 to 72 hours later.

TREATMENT:

EMERGENCY MEDICAL RESPONSE:

1. Remove the person from the source of exposure.
2. Place their hands beneath your armpits to warm them up.
3. Blow your warm, moist breath across them.
4. Put the affected area into contact with a warm object, such as holding hands above the heat of a stove or wrapping hands around a warm cup of tea or coffee. Do NOT burn them!

HOMEOPATHIC:

1. **Agaricus Muscarius 30C**, one dose every 15 minutes. Up to six doses.
2. **Petroleum 30C**, one dose every 15 minutes. Up to six doses.
3. **Laurocerasus 30C**, one dose every 15 minutes. Up to six doses.

NOTES _____

_____

_____

_____

_____

★HEAD INJURIES★

DEFINITION: All head injuries can be life threatening. Seventy percent of car accidents involve head injuries. Along with this, there can also be neck or spinal cord injury. The skull is composed of bones that protect our brain from injury.

Many types of head injury are discussed here: fracture of the skull, bruise of the brain (concussion), epidural hematoma (bleeding outside the dura which is the covering around the brain and beneath the skull), subdural hematoma (bleeding that occurs beneath the dura but outside of the brain), or intracerebral hematoma (bleeding in the brain tissue itself). All of these are very serious conditions and need an emergency response as soon as possible.

SIGNS, SYMPTOMS & INDICATORS:

HEAD INJURY IN GENERAL:

1. Laceration or contusion (bruising) of the scalp. This may or may not be present—so do not be fooled if there is no seeming physical injury present.
2. Visible fracture or a deformity in the skull (can be a depression of the bones as well).
3. "Raccoon eyes" or "Battle's sign, " where both eyes are blackened or there is bruising or swelling behind the ear(s) (the mastoid process).
4. Cerebrospinal fluid leakage from the scalp, eyes, nose, or ears—this is a watery, clear to pinkish, translucent fluid—although it might be mixed with blood and you will not be able to tell the difference. If this happens, the dura or covering over the brain has been torn, combined with a fracture to the skull, allowing this liquid to escape.
5. Failure of the pupils to respond to light (one or both eyes). Usually, the pupil that is unresponsive or fixed and will not respond to light will correspond to the side of the brain that has sustained the injury. The pupil on the uninjured side will respond.
6. Unequal pupil size.
7. Loss of sensation or motor functions—numb or tingling feeling in a limb or part of the body, or they cannot move it.
8. A period of unconsciousness.
9. Amnesia (loss of memory).
10. Retrograde amnesia (they cannot recall the events just before the accident occurred).
11. Confusion.

12. Visual complaints: blurred vision, partial vision, or double vision.
13. Combative or abnormal behavior.
14. Nausea/vomiting.
15. Dizziness.
16. Headache.

OTHER POSSIBLE SYMPTOMS:
1. Convulsions due to a buildup of fluid/blood within the skull that is pressing in on the brain tissue.
2. Cyanosis—the skin turns blue-gray—means that the person is not receiving enough oxygen due to the injury. It may mean that fluid buildup is placing pressure on the brain. They may have a blue color to their nail beds or around their mouth.
3. Physical weakness. Usually associated with a concussion, but may be seen with any other type of head injury as well.
4. Unusually sleepy after the head injury. At night, awaken the injured person every 4 hours.
5. Cannot keep their balance when they stand or walk.
6. Soreness along the spinal column/back area.

TREATMENT:

EMERGENCY MEDICAL RESPONSE:
1. Do NOT move the victim.
2. Make sure they are breathing. If not, administer CPR.
3. Do not move or elevate the head or neck region. Do not elevate the legs.
4. Try to keep the entire body stable—do not move them! However, if you must move them, use a log roll: Roll the victim toward you without moving head, neck, or back out of a straight line, as if they were a log. It takes one person to stabilize neck/head and the second person to pull at the arm/hip area to roll them. See page 16 for illustration. Treat for Shock, page 140.

HOMEOPATHIC: Consult with a homeopath after they have seen an MD.
1. **Arnica Montana 30C**, every 15 minutes, up to six doses. If unconscious place a drop of it on inside of wrist and rub it in.
2. **Helleborus 30C**, give with approval of homeopath, one dose.

Cerebral Hematoma: Epidural or Subdural Symptoms

DEFINITION: A hematoma is a contusion (bruising) to the brain—there is bleeding and swelling inside the brain. If it is bleeding between the skull and the dura, it is known as an epidural hematoma. If it is bleeding beneath the dura and directly into the brain, it is a subdural hematoma. This can put pressure on the brain stem at the back of the neck and the person's blood pressure goes up and pulse goes down. There can be serious respiratory problems. They have specific symptoms:

SIGNS, SYMPTOMS & INDICATORS:

1. Level of consciousness is the most important indicator. It may be altered.
2. Dizziness.
3. Headache.
4. Look at their pupils. A bruise or blow to the head will dilate one pupil and the other pupil will be fine.
5. Paralysis.
6. Projectile vomiting—extreme force; across the room.
7. Blood pressure goes UP.
8. Pulse rate goes DOWN.
9. Vision irregularities.
10. Irregular breathing or difficulty breathing. They may get into Kussmaul's Respiration (deep sighing breathing) or Cheyne-Stokes Respiration (person's breathing gets less and less deep, then quits, and then they take a deep breath and then it goes back into the Kussmaul's type of breathing).

TREATMENT:

EMERGENCY MEDICAL RESPONSE:
1. Do NOT move the victim.
2. Make sure they are breathing. If not, administer CPR.
3. Do not move or elevate the head or neck region. Do not elevate the legs.
4. Try to keep the entire body stable—do not move them! However, if you must move them use a log roll: Roll the victim toward you without moving head, neck, or back out of a straight line, as if they were a log. It takes one person to stabilize the neck/head and the second person to pull at the arm/hip area to roll them. Treat for Shock, page 140.

HOMEOPATHIC: Consult with a homeopath after an MD is seen.
1. **Arnica Montana 30C**, every 15 minutes, up to six doses. If unconscious place a drop of it on inside of wrist and rub it in.
2. **Helleborus 30C**. Give with approval of homeopath, one dose.

Intracranial Bleeding

DEFINITION: Known as an intracranial hematoma, it is the laceration of a blood vessel inside the brain or the meninges (the three layers of tissue that envelop the brain and spinal cord). There are three types: epidural hematoma, subdural hematoma, and intracerebral hematoma. (See Definition of Head Injuries.) This type of injury is swift moving, and every minute counts. Call 911 right away.

SIGNS, SYMPTOMS & INDICATORS:

1. Progressive loss of brain functions.
2. Death if not treated.
3. Deterioration is rapid and there are numerous neurological signs (paralysis, weakness, confusion, etc.).

TREATMENT:

EMERGENCY MEDICAL RESPONSE:
1. Do NOT move the person.
2. Make sure they are breathing. If not, perform CPR.
3. Do not move or elevate the head or neck. Do not elevate the legs.
4. Try to keep the entire body stable—do not move them! However, if you must move them it takes two, preferably three people for this maneuver, known as a log roll. Roll the person toward you without moving their head, neck, or back out of a straight line, as if they were a log. It takes one person to stabilize the neck/head and the second and/or third person to pull at the arm/hip and then the knee/ankle area, to roll them over in one fluid, stable motion. See page 16 for illustration. Treat for Shock, page 140.

HOMEOPATHIC: Consult a homeopath immediately.
1. **Arnica Montana 30C**, one dose every 15 minutes. Up to six doses. If unconscious, place a drop of the dilution on inside of wrist and rub in. Later, after stabilized …
2. **Helleborus 30C**. Consult with a homeopath first.

NOTES _____

_____

_____

★HEART ATTACK—GENERAL★

SIGNS, SYMPTOMS & INDICATORS:

1. "Crushing" chest pain, like a band around the chest.
2. Pressure or pain in the neck and up into the left or right jaw region.
3. Sweaty (shock).
4. Pale/ashen/gray color to face.
5. Stomach nausea which may be called "indigestion."
6. Shortness of breath. "Weight" or "pressure" in chest.
7. Pain radiates into the left or right arm—usually left because it is usually the LEFT ventricle of the heart that is involved.

TREATMENT:

EMERGENCY MEDICAL RESPONSE:

1. The heart is pumping fast. They need oxygen and they are sweaty. If they have oxygen nearby, administer it to them.
2. Have them sit down. If the pain goes away—call their doctor and find out what is going on. If the pain does NOT go away in **2 minutes**, call 911.

HOMEOPATHIC: Consult a homeopath for follow-up treatment.

1. **Aconitum Napellus 30C**, one dose every 15 minutes. Up to six doses.
2. **Cactus Grandiflorus 30C**, one dose every 15 minutes. Up to six doses.
3. **Ignatia Amara 30C** for panic/hysteria. One dose every 15 minutes. Up to six doses.

NOTES _____

_____

_____

_____

_____

Acute Myocardial Infarction

DEFINITION: A blood clot obstructs the left coronary artery of the heart and prevents blood from reaching the left (or right) ventricle. Plaque/cholesterol narrows the coronary artery and interferes with its ability to deliver blood and oxygen to the heart. Blockage of the coronary artery is called an occlusion (blockage). It signifies inadequate blood flow to the heart muscle.

SIGNS, SYMPTOMS & INDICATORS:

1. Pain is usually felt beneath the breastbone. It can radiate to the jaw (either side), to the arms (especially the left arm), or to the epigastrium (upper-middle region of the abdomen). It may go through the back to the digestive region. The pain won't necessarily go to all of these places.
2. Shortness of breath.
3. Nausea.
4. Sweating.
5. Squeezing sensation or tightness in the chest. They may say it feels like a belt tightening around them. It can also be felt as a crushing sensation or pressure in the chest.
6. Difficulty breathing.
7. Face has a pale or grayish look to it.
8. Blood pressure changes.
9. Heart rate is slow or fast or irregular. Heart palpitations.
10. They may or may not have pulmonary edema (swelling) in hands, feet, or ankles.
11. Pain lasts longer than 30 minutes.
12. It is not related to physical exertion, nor is it relieved by nitroglycerin tablets/patch/spray.
13. They may faint.
14. Extreme, sudden weakness; they cannot walk or stand.

TREATMENT:

EMERGENCY MEDICAL RESPONSE:
1. Reassure the person and calm them.
2. Try to get their medical history.
3. Position the person comfortably (usually sitting up and well supported).
4. Be prepared to perform CPR if necessary.
5. Treat for shock. (See Cardiogenic Shock, page 141.)

OTHER:
  1. Sometimes coughing will stop the heart from fibrillation (quivering, rapid heartbeats) and start it beating again. If it goes into fibrillation again, cough again. Keep person coughing as needed, until 911 help arrives.

HOMEOPATHIC: Consult a homeopath as soon after the attack as possible for follow-up treatment.
  1. **Cactus Grandiflorus 30C**, one dose every 15 minutes, as needed for crushing pain in chest, nausea, sweating, weakness, or fainting. Up to six doses.
  2. If there is a pending sense of doom heightened above all else, use **Aconitum Napellus 30C**, one dose every 15 minutes as needed. Up to six doses.
  3. If they show air hunger, a need for oxygen above all else, **Carbo Vegetabilis 30C**, one dose every 15 minutes as needed. Up to six doses.

NOTES _____

_____

_____

_____

_____

★HEART OPERATIONS★
PACEMAKERS

DEFINITION: Pacemaker is not working correctly.

SIGNS, SYMPTOMS & INDICATORS:

1. Fainting.
2. Dizziness.
3. Weakness.
4. Pulse slow—35 to 45 and irregular.

TREATMENT:

EMERGENCY MEDICAL RESPONSE:

1. Call 911. They will transport the person to the hospital because repair of the problem may require an operation.

HOMEOPATHIC:

1. **Aconitum Napellus 30C**, one dose every 15 minutes until their panic/hysteria disappears. Up to six doses.

NOTES _____

_____

_____

_____

_____

★HEAT CRAMPS★

See: Dehydration

DEFINITION: This happens to a person who goes outdoors and exercises too hard and long, especially in the heat; painful muscle spasms occur. Electrolytes are lost from the cells and dehydration may also play a role in the muscle cramping. Usually the legs and abdomen are involved.

SIGNS, SYMPTOMS & INDICATORS:

1. Cramping in the legs, hands, or feet.
2. Cramping in the abdomen.
3. Sweaty skin or cool, dry skin.
4. Severe pain.
5. Vital signs are normal.

TREATMENT:

EMERGENCY MEDICAL RESPONSE:
1. Drink fluids if conscious and alert. Gatorade, if available.
2. Get the person into the shade and out of the sunlight.
3. Loosen any tight clothing.
4. Rest the cramping muscles, massage the muscles, or stretch them.

HOMEOPATHIC:
1. **Belladonna 30C**, one dose every 15 minutes. Up to six doses.
2. Drink plenty of fluids.

NOTES

★HEAT EXHAUSTION★

See: Dehydration

DEFINITION: Referred to as heat prostration or heat collapse, it occurs when the body loses too much water via sweating. It can happen in hot or cold weather. Loss of liquids occurs faster than replacement.

SIGNS, SYMPTOMS & INDICATORS:

1. Skin cool and clammy.
2. Face gray or pale looking.
3. Nausea.
4. Headache.
5. Dizzy, weak, or faint feeling.
6. Pulse is rapid.
7. Blood pressure is normal.
8. Weakness.

TREATMENT:

EMERGENCY MEDICAL RESPONSE:
1. Treat for mild Shock, page 140. Person should lie on their back with feet elevated.
2. Loosen any tight clothing.
3. Move to shade or a cool environment (air conditioned car or house).
4. If conscious, give liquids.
5. If not recovered within 30 minutes, call 911.

HOMEOPATHIC:
1. **Belladonna 30C**, one dose every 15 minutes. Up to six doses.
2. **Glonoine 30C**, one dose every 15 minutes. Up to six doses.

NOTES _____

_____

_____

_____

_____

★HEAT STROKE★

See: Dehydration

DEFINITION: Also known as sun stroke, this can be potentially life threatening if not dealt with quickly. It occurs when the body is subject to more heat than it can handle and the normal mechanisms for getting rid of the excess heat are overwhelmed. Untreated heat stroke will result in death. The body temperature rises rapidly and the core temperature rises, which affects all the vital organs. The person's level of consciousness rapidly decreases.

SIGNS, SYMPTOMS & INDICATORS:

1. Hot, dry skin.
2. Change in behavior or bizarre behavior.
3. Pulse rapid and strong.
4. Blood pressure decreasing.
5. Level of consciousness varies to unconsciousness.
6. Coma.

TREATMENT:

EMERGENCY MEDICAL RESPONSE:
1. Get the person out of the hot environment and into the shade.
2. Get the person cooled off—take off their clothes, but they may need a light sheet to keep from getting chilled later.
3. Cover them with wet towels or sheet.
4. Fan them with whatever you have available.
5. Protect their airway. Perform CPR if necessary.
6. Call 911. If there is no way to contact them, transport the person immediately to a hospital and set the car air conditioning on high.

HOMEOPATHIC: Consult a homeopath for follow-up treatment.
1. Follow all procedures above and …
2. **Glonoine 30C**, one dose every 15 minutes. Up to six doses.
3. **Belladonna 30C**, one dose every 15 minutes. Up to six doses.

NOTES _____

_____

_____

_____

_____

★HIP FRACTURE★

DEFINITION: This is a common injury for the elderly and when it occurs, they think they've "broken their hip." In reality, it usually involves the proximal or top of the femur or thigh bone. The break or fracture is through the neck of the femur but the person will THINK that it is their hip and only x-rays will reveal the true area of the fracture.

SIGNS, SYMPTOMS & INDICATORS:

1. The injured person will lie with their broken leg shortened and displaced. The foot is pointed out, or rotated externally from its normal position. The toe will point away from the person's body— so this is your key to recognize the type of fracture it is.
2. They are unable to walk or move that leg due to severe pain.
3. There will be pain in the hip region or the inner area of the thigh.
4. There may also be 'referred' pain in the knee of the affected leg.

TREATMENT:

EMERGENCY MEDICAL RESPONSE:
1. Keep the person as calm as possible until help arrives.
2. Treat for Shock, page 140.
3. Cover all wounds with dressings.
4. Do NOT replace protruding bone(s).
5. If no 911 help is nearby, use a pillow or pillows around the fracture as a splint, tape it, and pad the splint(s) with a blanket or other material to fill in the voids, particularly if you use wood for splint material. If a leg is involved, "splint" the broken leg to the good leg. Place a blanket or material between the legs to stabilize, then tape them together.
6. It is important to leave the injured leg in its deformed position. Do NOT try to pull, twist, or move it in any way.
7. Splint above and below the joint.

HOMEOPATHIC: Consult a homeopath for follow-up treatment.

1. Give **Arnica Montana 30C**, one dose every 15 minutes until shock is stabilized and for muscle/tissue damage/bleeding/shock symptoms. If no 911 help is nearby, continue to give once an hour if they are shocky. Up to eight doses or until you can reach a medical facility. If that does not stabilize their shock, go to **Aconitum Napellus 30C**, one dose every 15 minutes until shock is stabilized and for muscle/tissue damage/bleeding/shock symptoms. If no 911 help is nearby, continue to give once an hour if they are shocky. Up to eight doses or until you can reach a medical facility.

2. **Arnica Montana 30C,** for swelling and bruising afterward. Consult a homeopath first.
3. **Symphytum 30C,** restores bone growth and knitting at optimum speed. Consult a homeopath first.
4. **Calcarea Phosphorica 30C** if fracture does not heal in a reasonable amount of time, usually 8 weeks. Consult a homeopath first.
5. One week afterward: **Bellis Perennis 30C.** Consult a homeopath first.

NOTES _____

_____

_____

_____

_____

★HYPERVENTILATION★

DEFINITION: These symptoms are usually brought on by emotional stress/hysteria/excitement or anxiety.

SIGNS, SYMPTOMS & INDICATORS:

1. Some kind of psychological stress is present.
2. Breathing is very fast and shallow.
3. Fainting.
4. Stabbing pain in the chest (they think they're having a heart attack).
5. Dizziness.
6. Cramping in the fingers and toes—later in the legs and arms.
7. Numbness or tingling in the fingers and toes.

TREATMENT:

EMERGENCY MEDICAL RESPONSE:

1. Do NOT use a paper bag to blow into.
2. Instead, be calm, supportive, and keep your voice low. Speak to them and calm them down, stay with them and talk them out of it. Breathe with them.
3. Have them breathe in through their nostrils, and blow out through their pursed lips—do this in sync with them.

HOMEOPATHIC:

NOTE: If they have fainted, do NOT give anything by mouth. If you have the homeopathic dilution, rub one drop on inside of one wrist every 5 minutes. If you have none, use Bach Rescue Remedy and rub one drop on inside of wrist every 5 minutes until they regain consciousness.

1. **Aconitum Napellus 30C**, one dose every 15 minutes. Up to six doses.
2. **Ignatia Amara 30C**, one dose every 15 minutes. Up to six doses.
3. **Moschus 30C**, one dose every 15 minutes. Up to six doses.

SEE: Shortness of Breath (Dyspnea).

NOTES _____

_____

_____

_____

_____

★HYPOTHERMIA★

See: Frostnip, Frostbite (Superficial), and Frostbite (Deep)

DEFINITION: The core temperature of the body is lowered by being out too long in cold weather with or without adequate clothing and protection. There are five general stages of hypothermia where the core temperature of the body goes from 95 degrees F to below 78 degrees F. Frost nip, superficial frost bite, and deep frost bite are covered under their separate names. The general symptoms of hypothermia are as follows:

SIGNS, SYMPTOMS & INDICATORS:

1. Shivering.
2. Fine muscle coordination (such as writing ability) decreases.
3. Gross motor muscle coordination decreases; they have trouble walking and they may stagger.
4. Their breathing slows.
5. Pulse is weak and decreasing to slow.
6. Muscles are stiff.

TREATMENT:

EMERGENCY MEDICAL RESPONSE:
1. If no breathing and/or pulse, perform CPR.
2. Prevent further heat loss but do not try to rewarm the person.
3. Remove all wet clothing, cover with a blanket, and keep them at 70 degrees F.
4. If unconscious, gently palpate the carotid artery for one minute to check for a pulse.
5. Handle the person VERY gently—do not bump them.
6. When calling 911, ask for instructions on what else to do until medical help arrives.

HOMEOPATHIC: Consult homeopath for follow-up treatment.
1. **Laurocerasus 30C**, one dose every 15 minutes, for collapse due to coldness. Up to six doses.

NOTES _____

_____

_____

_____

_____

★IMPALED OBJECTS★

DEFINITION: A puncture type of wound where the object remains in the body. There can be blood loss and infection. For example, it could be an impaled knife, stick, or metal object.

SIGNS, SYMPTOMS & INDICATORS:

1. Tenderness.
2. Swelling.
3. Bruising.
4. Deformity.
5. Loss of function.

TREATMENT:

EMERGENCY MEDICAL RESPONSE:
1. **Safety for yourself first—evaluate all possible dangers. Make sure there are none—otherwise, you become a victim too.**
2. Keep the person as calm as possible. Do not remove impaled object.
3. Do not move the person unless they are in immediate danger (car fire, out in the middle of a highway, etc.)
4. Perform CPR if necessary.
5. Stabilize the impaled object with a bulky dressing around it—further movement will increase damage to soft tissue.
6. Control the bleeding with more compresses around it, or use indirect pressure of either the femoral or brachial artery to slow the hemorrhaging at the injury site. (See Bleeding, page 38.)
7. Protect wound from further damage—have the person lie quietly.
8. Prevent further contamination of the wound by using clean, dry, sterile dressings.

HOMEOPATHIC: Consult a homeopath for follow-up treatment.
IF AUTO OR TRAUMA ACCIDENT:
1. **Arnica Montana 30C**, one dose every 15 minutes for hemorrhage/shock/tissue damage. Up to six doses.
2. **Aconitum Napellus 30C**, one dose every 15 minutes if shock comes back within an hour after the accident. This is for deeply rooted shock. If shock is still present, consult a homeopath as soon as possible.
3. **Pyrogenium 30C** for sepsis, blood poisoning that occurs after impaled object is removed and the person is on antibiotics. With approval of their homeopath, first.

4. **Hypericum 30C**, once a day for 4 days, if there is nerve injury along with impalement. Give after object is removed. With approval of their homeopath, first.
5. **Ledum 30C**, one dose, shortly after object is removed. Give after coming out of post-surgical anesthesia.

OTHER LESS TRAUMATIC ACCIDENTS:

1. **Arnica Montana 30C**, one dose every 15 minutes. Up to six doses.
2. **Bellis Perennis 30C**, if swelling/bruising is not completely gone after administration of **Arnica Montana**. Consult a homeopath first.

EYE INJURY:

1. **Aconitum Napellus 30C**, one dose every 15 minutes, after impaled object is removed and until swelling is reduced and pain is gone. Up to six doses.
2. If **Aconitum Napellus** does not stop symptoms completely, go to …
3. **Symphytum 30C**, one dose once an hour. Up to six doses.

NOTES _____

_____

_____

_____

_____

★INTERNAL INJURIES★

See: Abdominal Injuries, Head Injuries, and Chest Injuries

DEFINITION: An injury that is not visible—to the head, chest, or abdominal area. There may be not only laceration of an organ, but also a tearing open of one accompanied by severe bleeding or hemorrhage.

EMERGENCY MEDICAL RESPONSE:

1. Make sure the person is breathing and has a pulse—if not, call 911 and begin CPR.
2. Perform a Primary Survey (page 9).
3. If airway, breathing, and pulse are stable, perform a Secondary Survey (page 12). If there are any outer signs of bleeding, place a compress with direct pressure upon the injury. NOTE: Do not turn them over if you suspect spinal injury.
4. Feel under clothes for any sticky fluid (blood).
5. If you find a wound, and if you have a pair of scissors, cut away the clothing in that area and place a compress on it with direct pressure.
6. If there is no external bleeding, examine the person from head to toe. (See How to Perform a Primary and Secondary Survey of the person, page 9.) If the person is conscious, ask them where it hurts.
7. Look for any sign of deformity (swelling, bruising, or unusual hardness of skin where there should be softness).

SEE: Specific type of injury and how to respond further to it, plus the appropriate homeopathic remedies for it.

NOTES _____

_____

_____

_____

_____

★KNEE INJURY★

SIGNS, SYMPTOMS & INDICATORS:

1. Swelling at the site.
2. Pain in the affected joint area.
3. Bruising.
4. Point of tenderness if pressed gently with index finger.

TREATMENT:

EMERGENCY MEDICAL RESPONSE:

1. Splint above and below it.
2. Keep weight off of it.
3. **RICE** therapy: Rest, Ice, Compression and Elevation.
   a. First 1 or 2 days allow the area to rest completely (or more, depending upon what the doctor says). Then exercise the joint gently without putting weight on it. Person may need physical therapy, depending upon the severity. See a doctor for further instructions, first.
   b. Ice pack or bag of frozen vegetables (place a towel between the ice bag and skin) and either hold it on or use an elastic bandage. Continue ice treatment for 20 minutes at 1 or 2 hour intervals if awake. After 24 hours, switch to heat and soak joint in hot (not burning) water whenever possible for 15 minutes at a time, every 2 hours.
   c. Compression. Use an elastic bandage around the injured area.
   d. Elevate the extremity. Do this while sleeping; also place a small pillow beneath the area so the excess fluid can drain out of the area instead of collecting there overnight.

HOMEOPATHIC:

1. **Ruta Graveolens 30C**, one dose every 15 minutes, if it is WORSE with continued movement. Up to six doses.
2. **Rhus Toxicodendron 30C**, one dose every 15 minutes, if it is BETTER with movement. Up to six doses.
3. **Bellis Perennis 30C**, one dose every 15 minutes, if neither of the above remedies are working.
4. **Symphytum 30C**, helps to heal ligaments sooner and faster. Consult a homeopath about this first.

NOTES _____

_____

_____

★LIGHTNING STRIKE★

DEFINITION: A thousand people are struck by lightning each year and 200 of them die from it. Lightning contains up to 50 million volts of electricity and may be 50,000 degrees F. People can receive one of the following: A direct strike (the worst type of injury), a flash over (lightning travels over the surface of the person to the ground and they are standing in a wet area), a side flash (lightning hits nearby and 'splashes' through the air to strike the person), and a stride potential (lightning strikes the ground, travels up one leg of the person, goes down the other leg, and dissipates into the ground).

A lightning strike may cause deep tissue injury and does cause the heart to stop beating and the person to stop breathing. CPR is often needed immediately in these cases. You also have to deal with blunt trauma to the person where the bolt struck them, unconsciousness, potential paralysis (which may or may not be permanent), amnesia, and mental confusion.

FURTHER PREVENTION OF A LIGHTNING STRIKE:

1. Get out of the water, or away from it if you are boating, fishing, or swimming.
2. Stay away from umbrellas, golf clubs, tent poles, metal fences, baseball backstops, or fishing poles, all of which conduct electricity.
3. Do not stand out in the open, on top of a hill/mountain/ridge, in any kind of natural land depression, or at the mouth of a cave.
4. Do not hold a telephone and be talking on it, be in a bath or taking a shower, be ironing clothes, or be around any electrical appliance. Shut off your computer and unplug it.
5. Do not stand near any tall object (tree, pole, or tower) of any kind.
6. If you have no way of reaching shelter, squat down (try to find a dry area, not a wet one), facing downhill. Make yourself as small a target as possible to lightning. Keep your hands out of contact with the ground. If you have a metal backpack frame, get rid of it and any sleeping gear, including foam pads.
7. If there are several people with you, spread them out to lessen the possibility of lightning striking them as a group.

DO

1. Get into a building, a car (not a convertible or open sport utility type), a deep cave, or a large stand of trees that are shorter and of more uniform size.

TREATMENT:

EMERGENCY MEDICAL RESPONSE:

1. Get the person or people out of danger from another lightning strike because lightning WILL strike twice in the same place. Move anything such as an umbrella or golf club away from the individual and yourself.
2. Treat for Shock, page 140.

HOMEOPATHIC:

NOTE: If wrists have been burned, and patient is unconscious, do NOT place homeopathic dilution drop on wrist. Place drop behind the ear (if not burned) and gently rub into the skin. If person is conscious, give one drop in their mouth instead.

1. If unconscious, but breathing, **Opium 30C**, once every 15 minutes. Up to six doses.
2. Get a professional homeopath to see the person as soon as possible after the accident.
3. If conscious but shocky, **Aconitum Napellus 30C**, once every 15 minutes. Up to six doses.

NOTES _____

_____

_____

_____

_____

★LYME DISEASE★

SEE: Tick Bites and Rocky Mountain Spotted Fever

DEFINITION: Ticks carry the bacteria *Borrelia burgdorferi*, a newly discovered spirochete. The white-footed mouse is the primary reservoir for this tick. Deer are a preferred host, but so are other mammals, especially dogs. This disease was discovered in 1975 in Lyme, Connecticut. It has since appeared in 43 states. It usually occurs in summer and early fall. Children and young adults who live in heavily wooded areas are bitten the most. Incubation is 3 to 32 days. It is a PAINLESS bite. It travels through the lymph system and 85% of these people get arthritis symptoms from it.

PRECAUTIONS: Tick bites are painless and you will not feel them attach to you, so do the following:
1. Wear light-colored clothing so you can spot the dark brown tick.
2. Tuck your pant cuffs into your socks.
3. Examine yourself or your children several times.
4. Ticks like warm, moist parts of the body or folds of skin—check all of these areas carefully. They also like to live in hair—so check the scalp, under the arms, and in the genital area as well.
5. Pets should be examined thoroughly when they get home.

SIGNS, SYMPTOMS & INDICATORS:

1. The bite is painless.
2. A red spot on the skin appears where the person was bitten; 75% of the people develop lesions; 50% develop a number of red spots with white centers over much of their body.
3. Flu-like symptoms appear a few days after the lesions: fatigue, chill, fever, headache, stiff neck, pain, and arthritis-like symptoms (bones and joints ache).
4. Nausea or vomiting.
5. Sore throat.
6. Lymph glands are swollen in neck, beneath armpits, and in the groin region.
7. Backache.
8. Many of these symptoms come and go, appear and disappear intermittently and are changeable.
9. The weakness and fatigue may come and go, but stays for weeks at a time afterward.
10. Arthritis symptoms appear within weeks or months of onset, or may not appear up to 2 years after the initial bite. Knees are most affected.

11. Baker's cysts (large lumps under the skin, anywhere on the body) may form and rupture. They also come and go and are intermittent.

TREATMENT:

EMERGENCY MEDICAL RESPONSE:

1. Remove the tick with tweezers by pulling straight out of the skin. Do not worry if the head of the tick remains. It is more important to remove the body, which harbors the bacteria. See your physician right away.
2. Paint area with a disinfectant.
3. Save the tick so it can be identified. Do NOT handle the tick with your fingers! Wear rubber or latex gloves.

HOMEOPATHIC: Consult a homeopath for follow-up treatment.

AFTER REMOVING THE TICK:

1. **Rhus Toxicodendron 30C**, one dose an hour. Up to six doses.
2. **Pyrogenium 30C**, if bite site becomes septic (blood poisoning). See MD and homeopath right away.
3. **Ledum 30C**, one dose every hour IF bite site is COLD to your touch.

NOTES _____

_____

_____

_____

_____

★MARINE ANIMAL STINGS★

DEFINITION: A bite from a jellyfish or a sting ray, or stepping on a sea urchin. These are covered in separate categories here in alphabetical order:

Anemones, Corals, Jellyfish, Hydras & Portuguese Man-o-War

SIGNS, SYMPTOMS & INDICATORS:

1. Intense burning sensation of skin around sting.
2. Red, raised welt that develops rapidly.
3. Weakness.
4. Headache.
5. Muscle pain.
6. Spasms.
7. Tearing eyes.
8. Nasal discharge.
9. Sweating.
10. Changes in pulse rate.
11. Chest pain that increases with breathing.

TREATMENT:

EMERGENCY MEDICAL RESPONSE:
1. Remove the person from the water.
2. Pour rubbing alcohol on the affected area.
3. Sprinkle the area with meat tenderizer.
4. Dust with talcum powder afterward.

NOTE: The alcohol fixes or denatures the toxin and the meat tenderizer destroys it.

HOMEOPATHIC:
1. **Apis Mellifica 30C**, one dose every 15 minutes. Up to six doses.
2. **Hypericum Tincture**—dilute 1:10 (1 teaspoon per quart of water) and wash the area three times daily for 2 days.
3. **Lachesis 30C**, one dose every 15 minutes. Up to six doses.

Cone Shells, Urchins, Spiny Fish (Catfish, Toad or Oyster Fish) & Stingrays—Puncture Wounds

SIGNS, SYMPTOMS & INDICATORS:

1. Puncture wound site is highly painful.

TREATMENT:

EMERGENCY MEDICAL RESPONSE:

1. Wash off with sea water at hand.
2. Attempt to remove the stinger from the wound if it is seen in the wound. If not, do not do anything.
3. Submerge extremity in as hot a water as they can stand for 30 to 90 minutes. (Do NOT burn them!)
4. Watch for allergic reaction. (See Allergic Reaction, page 25.)

NOTE: The toxins are destroyed by hot water. Do NOT use water so hot that it scalds the person. The pain in the wound may make the skin around it less sensitive to heat than normal, so be very watchful of this.

HOMEOPATHIC:

1. **Apis Mellifica 30C**, one dose every 15 minutes. Up to six doses.
2. **Hypericum Tincture**—dilute 1:10 (or 1 teaspoon per quart of water) and wash the area three times daily for 2 days.
3. **Ledum 30C**, one dose every 15 minutes. Up to six doses.

NOTES _____

_____

_____

_____

_____

★NOSEBLEED★

DEFINITION: Known as "Epistaxis," this is a common emergency in the home. Sometimes, enough blood can be lost to cause shock; the blood coming from the nose is small in comparison to what is being swallowed. If a person swallows enough blood, they will vomit, which exacerbates the problem. The reasons for the nosebleed need to be understood so that you know whether or not to call 911.

REASONS FOR NOSEBLEEDS:

1. Person has sustained a fractured skull or head injury.
2. Injuries to the face (or to the nose).
3. Sinus infections, overuse of nasal sprays or drops, dried or cracked mucosa lining within the nostrils (from low humidity or desert-like conditions), or other abnormalities within the nasal passage (such as polyps usually seen on a person with allergies).
4. High blood pressure.
5. Having a bleeder's disease (hemophilia).

TREATMENT:

EMERGENCY MEDICAL RESPONSE:

1. If the person is unconscious, and/or bleeding, call 911.
2. If you have a blood pressure cuff and stethoscope, take the person's blood pressure first. Ask them if they are on high blood pressure medication. If they are, ask if they are taking it on a regular basis. If blood pressure is high (over 140/90 for an adult) then you know what is causing the nosebleed. They should notify their MD of the situation. See a homeopath for constitutional treatment to cure the high blood pressure symptoms.
3. If the person is conscious, ask the above questions in 'reasons for nosebleeds' and see if you can identify what is causing it.
4. Apply pressure just below the bony ridge of the nose, to halt the bleeding. Do this for at least 10 to 15 minutes.
5. Have the person sitting up and leaning slightly forward during this time.
6. Or, place a 4 x 4 gauze bandage, rolled up, between the upper lip and gum of the person. Have them press against it with their fingers to slow blood supply.
7. Apply ice over the nose.
8. It will take 15 minutes, sometimes, to halt it—do not remove the pressure from the nose once you've applied your fingers to it, during this time frame.

HOMEOPATHIC:

1. **Phosphorus 30C**, one dose, will usually halt most types of nosebleeds within 5 minutes of taking it. A second dose may be used, if necessary.

2. **Arnica Montana 30C**, one dose every 15 minutes, if the person has sustained a blow to the face or nose. Up to six doses.

3. If the nosebleed is due to high blood pressure, have them call their doctor and then seek a professional homeopath as soon as possible after the incident.

NOTES _____

_____

_____

_____

_____

★OPEN WOUND★

DEFINITION: Skin that is cut by a penetrating object.

SIGNS, SYMPTOMS & INDICATORS:

1. Tenderness.
2. Swelling.
3. Bruising.
4. Deformity.
5. Loss of function.

TREATMENT:

EMERGENCY MEDICAL RESPONSE:

1. **Safety for yourself first—evaluate all possible dangers. Make sure there are none—otherwise, you become a victim, too.**
2. Place a compress over the wound site and apply direct pressure to it. If it is an eye injury, apply **NO** pressure. Cover with a dressing only.
3. Treat for Shock, page 140.
4. Ask, "What happened?" and "Where do you hurt?"
5. If bleeding does not stop, apply indirect pressure on either brachial (under arm) artery or femoral artery (where thigh attaches to the trunk of the body). See Bleeding, page 38.

HOMEOPATHIC:

IF AUTO OR TRAUMA ACCIDENT:

1. **Arnica Montana 30C**, one dose every 15 minutes for hemorrhage/shock/tissue damage. Up to six doses.
2. **Aconitum Napellus 30C**, one dose every 15 minutes, if shock comes back within an hour of the accident.
3. **Pyrogenium 30C**, for sepsis, blood poisoning that occurs even though an antibiotic is being used. Consult a homeopath first.
4. **Hypericum 30C**, if there is nerve injury along with impalement. Consult a homeopath first.
5. **Calendula Tincture**—use as a sterilizing wash. Dilute 1:10 with water (1 teaspoon per quart of water). Wash area three times daily for 2 days. NEVER use on puncture wounds. Use **Hypericum Tincture** 1:10, instead.

OTHER LESS TRAUMATIC ACCIDENTS:

1. **Arnica Montana 30C**, one dose every 15 minutes for hemorrhage/shock/tissue damage. Up to six doses.
2. **Bellis Perennis 30C**, if swelling/bruising is not completely gone after giving **Arnica Montana**. Consult a homeopath first.

EYE INJURY:

1. **Aconitum Napellus 30C**, one dose every 15 minutes until swelling is reduced and pain is gone. Up to six doses. If **Aconitum Napellus** does not stop it completely, go to ...

2. **Symphytum 30C**, one dose every 15 minutes. Up to six doses.

NOTES _____

_____

_____

_____

_____

★PLANT POISONING★

DEFINITION: Thousands of cases of plant poisoning occur each year, usually to young children. Many household plants are poisonous. Call your state Poison Center or Control for a list of these plants. The three types of physical disturbances caused by plants are covered individually here.

Circulatory Disturbance

DEFINITION: The person will show signs of circulatory collapse 30 to 50 minutes after eating the plant.

SIGNS, SYMPTOMS & INDICATORS:

1. Rapid, racing heartbeat.
2. Falling blood pressure.
3. Weakness.
4. Sweating.
5. Skin is cold, moist, and clammy feeling—they're going into shock—treat for Shock, page 140.

TREATMENT:

EMERGENCY MEDICAL RESPONSE: There is no known antidote for plant poisonings that cause circulatory collapse.
1. Call 911 and Poison Control.
2. Lay the person down and elevate their legs.
3. Perform CPR if necessary.
4. Induce vomiting with Syrup of Ipecac if the person is alert and conscious.
5. Pluck several leaves from the plant and put into a ziplock bag to give to 911 personnel for identification.
6. Collect vomitus and give to arriving medical personnel.

HOMEOPATHIC: Consult a homeopath for follow-up treatment.
1. Follow the above treatment.
2. **Digitalis 30C**, one dose every 15 minutes until stabilized. Up to six doses.
3. **Arsenicum Album 30C**, after having vomited with the use of Syrup of Ipecac. One dose every hour or until symptoms are gone. No more than six doses.

Gastrointestinal Disturbance

DEFINITION: These symptoms occur within 20–30 minutes of ingestion.

SIGNS, SYMPTOMS & INDICATORS:

1. Vomiting.
2. Diarrhea.
3. Cramps.
4. Difficulty speaking.
5. Irritation of mucous membranes and lining of stomach/mouth.
6. Difficulty swallowing.

TREATMENT:

EMERGENCY MEDICAL RESPONSE:

1. Call 911 and Poison Control immediately.
2. Maintain an open airway. Perform CPR if necessary.
3. Pluck several leaves from the plant and put into a ziplock bag to give to 911 personnel for identification.
4. Some people may take longer to show the symptoms. Do not induce vomiting.
5. Collect vomitus and give to arriving medical personnel.

HOMEOPATHIC:

1. Treat as above.
2. **Arsenicum Album 30C**, one dose every 15 minutes. If person vomits, repeat the remedy again, shortly afterward. Up to six doses.
3. May need **Formica Rufus 30C** for red, itching, burning mucosa surfaces—eyes, mouth, throat, etc.), once every 15 minutes until symptoms are relieved. Up to six doses.

Central Nervous System Disturbance

DEFINITION: This kind of plant poisoning can be lethal. Do not induce vomiting in any person who shows any signs of stupor or coma.

SIGNS, SYMPTOMS & INDICATORS:

1. Hyperactivity.
2. Depression.
3. Very excited.
4. Mental confusion.
5. Stupor.
6. Coma.

TREATMENT:

EMERGENCY MEDICAL RESPONSE:
1. Call 911 and Poison Control immediately.
2. Perform CPR if necessary.
3. Do not induce vomiting in a semiconscious or unconscious person.
4. Pluck several leaves from the plant and put into a ziplock bag to give to 911 personnel for identification.

HOMEOPATHIC:
1. **Tarantula Hispania 30C**, one dose every 15 minutes if hyperactive or excitable. Up to six doses.
2. **Opium 30C**, if depressed and in stupor or unconscious. If unconscious, rub one drop on the inner wrist. One dose every 15 minutes. Up to six doses.

Skin Irritants—Poison Oak/Ivy

DEFINITION: One of the most common forms of plant poisoning. Most people know of poison ivy and oak and have had a run-in with the sap or oil on these plants at some point in their lives.

SIGNS, SYMPTOMS & INDICATORS:

1. Redness of skin surface.
2. Blisters.
3. Itching.
4. Swelling.

TREATMENT:

EMERGENCY MEDICAL RESPONSE:
1. Thorough cleansing with soap and water. This treatment is most effective 30 to 60 minutes after coming into contact with poison.
2. Remove clothing that may have been affected.

HOMEOPATHIC:
1. Vigorously wash off the affected area with Fels Naptha soap.
2. If the poison symptoms appear hours or days after the cleansing …
3. **Rhus Toxicodendron 30C**. There are many other remedies in cases of poison oak/ivy, so a homeopath should be consulted.

NOTES _____

_____

_____

_____

★POISONING★

DEFINITION: There are many types of poisons and poisoning symptoms. Poisons can be inhaled, ingested, or contacted with one's skin. They can disturb the circulatory, gastrointestinal, or central nervous system. All are dangerous and potentially lethal. They are not all covered here. If you suspect poisoning, call your state's Poison Control phone number, plus 911.

GENERAL POISONING SYMPTOMS:

1. Nausea.
2. Vomiting.
3. Abdominal pain.
4. Diarrhea.
5. Dilation or constriction of the pupils.
6. Excessive salivation.
7. Sweating.
8. Difficulty breathing.
9. Cyanosis—blueness of the fingernail beds or around the mouth.
10. Depressed breathing.
11. Convulsions.
12. Unconsciousness.
13. Signs around the mouth such as burns, an odor on the breath, or stains.

TREATMENT:

EMERGENCY MEDICAL RESPONSE:

If the substance ingested is NOT an acid, alkali, or petroleum product, follow the steps below. If an acid, alkali, or petroleum product was ingested, dilute with milk or water, only, and do NOT induce vomiting. Call Poison Control immediately.

IF INGESTED POISON IS NOT AN ACID, ALKALI, OR PETROLEUM PRODUCT, DO THE FOLLOWING:

1. Call 911 and Poison Control.
2. Dilute poison with milk or water.
3. Use Syrup of Ipecac to induce vomiting if the person is conscious. If unconscious, do NOT give anything. For adults give a 30cc dose with two glasses of water. For children, give 15cc with two glasses of water. Wait 20 minutes. If the person does not vomit, give again in the same amounts.

<u>IF AN ACID, ALKALI, OR PETROLEUM PRODUCT WAS INGESTED,
DO THE FOLLOWING:</u>
1. Call 911 and Poison Control.
2. Use activated charcoal—50 to 100 grams must be ingested. This substance is made from 20% India ink and some people are allergic to the activated charcoal for this reason—so be watchful for an anaphylactic or allergic reaction.

SEE: Allergic Reaction, page 25.

Contact Poisons

DEFINITION: If you are working around any dry chemical substance and get it on your skin, there is a potential for poisoning because the skin is permeable and can absorb the dust or granules. Call Poison Control.

TREATMENT:

EMERGENCY MEDICAL RESPONSE:
1. Remove the irritating or corrosive substance as soon as possible by carefully dusting it off your skin. Make SURE that nobody, including you, inhales the substance—take precautions!
2. Remove all clothing.
3. Get into a shower and 'flood' the affected area for at least 15 to 20 minutes for ALKALIS and 5 minutes for ACIDS. Clean skin off with running water.
4. Wash the area off with soap and water.

HOMEOPATHIC: Consult a homeopath for follow-up treatment.
1. Perform the above procedures.
2. If any burning symptoms remain, **Arsenicum Album** 30C, one dose every 15 minutes. Up to six doses.
3. **Carbo Vegetabilis 30C**, one dose every 15 minutes, if the person is having trouble breathing. Up to six doses.

Inhaled Poisons

DEFINITION: Two common types of inhaled poisons are carbon monoxide from a car and chlorine from around a swimming pool. Farmers who open bags of insecticides and pesticides without proper masks and protection can also inhale deadly, poisonous materials. Call Poison Control immediately. See Chlorine Poisoning, page 133.

Chlorine Poisoning

DEFINITION: Working around a swimming pool can be a hazard, especially if you inhale the fumes of those green crystals that you put into your pool to keep it clean. Another source would be a hazardous material spill and the green cloud, which is indicative of chlorine, being inhaled by people downwind from the incident. This gas causes progressive lung damage and if caught in time, the person will require 2–3 days in intensive care to survive the incident.

SIGNS, SYMPTOMS & INDICATORS:

1. Severe respiratory irritation.
2. Severe eye irritation.
3. Epiglottis spasms in throat.
4. Coughing.
5. Choking.
6. Vomiting.
7. Pulmonary edema—fluid in the lungs.
8. Cyanosis.
9. Irritation to the throat that produces airway obstruction by swelling the tissue in that region.

TREATMENT:

EMERGENCY MEDICAL RESPONSE:
1. Protect yourself first. If possible remove the person from the contaminated area.
2. Perform CPR if necessary.

HOMEOPATHIC: Consult a homeopath for follow-up treatment.
1. **Arsenicum Album 30C**, one dose every 15 minutes until the person stabilizes. Up to six doses.
2. **Carbolicum Acidum 30C**, one dose every 15 minutes until the person stabilizes. Up to six doses.
3. **Opium 30C**, one dose every 5 minutes if person is found in a coma and CPR is not reviving them (continue CPR and) … have another person place one drop on inside of their wrist and rub it in.

NOTES _____

_____

_____

_____

★PUNCTURE WOUND★

See: Soft Tissue Injuries

DEFINITION: The wound that results from a stab with a knife, ice pick, or other pointed object, such as a bullet, splinter, or piece of glass.

SIGNS, SYMPTOMS & INDICATORS:

1. Usually very little bleeding involved.
2. Swelling.
3. Pain.

IF A GUNSHOT WOUND:

1. The entrance point is usually smaller than the exit point, which can be much larger.
2. Small-caliber bullets can deflect off bones and lodge in the organs.
3. Find out what caliber gun was used to help assess the amount of possible damage.

TREATMENT:

EMERGENCY MEDICAL RESPONSE:

1. Do NOT remove the object. Perform CPR if necessary.
2. Stabilize the impaled object with a bulky dressing around it—further movement will increase damage to soft tissue.
3. Control bleeding with more compresses around it, or use indirect pressure of either the femoral or brachial artery to slow the hemorrhaging at the injury site. (See Bleeding, page 38.)
4. Protect the wound from further damage—keep the person quiet.
5. Prevent further contamination of the wound by using clean, dry sterile dressings.

HOMEOPATHIC:

1. **Arnica Montana 30C**, one dose every 15 minutes. Up to six doses.

IF A MAJOR WOUND: Consult homeopath.

1. **Arnica Montana 30C**, one dose every 15 minutes. Up to six doses.
2. **Ledum 30C**, one dose every 15 minutes, if a puncture wound. Up to six doses.

IF A GUNSHOT WOUND: Consult homeopath.

1. **Arnica Montana 30C**, one dose every 15 minutes. Up to six doses.
2. **China 30C**, one dose every 15 minutes, for shock/excessive bleeding (internal or external). Up to six doses.

NOTES _____

★RIB FRACTURE★

SIGNS, SYMPTOMS & INDICATORS:

1. Point of tenderness—localized pain.
2. Deformity of a rib(s).
3. Chest wall may be bruised or lacerated.
4. Deep breathing, coughing, or movement is usually very painful.
5. Person tries to remain very still.
6. Person will take rapid, shallow breaths.
7. Person may lean toward the injured side.
8. Person will place a hand over the area to "splint" it or to try to ease the pain.
9. Pain in liver or spleen region—this is a rib lacerating the organ(s).

TREATMENT:

EMERGENCY MEDICAL RESPONSE:

1. Place a triangular bandage with a swathe on that arm to keep it supported and stabilized.

HOMEOPATHIC:

1. **Aconitum Napellus 30C**, one dose every 15 minutes. Up to six doses for the shock.
2. **Arnica Montana 30C**, one dose every 15 minutes. Up to six doses if bleeding or hemorrhaging is involved, along with shock.
3. **Symphytum 30C**, to speed healing of bone. Consult a homeopath before initiating.
4. **Ruta Graveolens 30C**, for multiple bone fractures and injury to muscles, tendons, or connective tissue. Consult a homeopath first before initiating.

NOTES _____

_____

_____

_____

_____

★ROCKY MOUNTAIN★ SPOTTED FEVER

See: Lyme Disease and Tick Bites

DEFINITION: This occurs 7 to 10 days after being bitten, although incubation can be 3 to 12 days. It can be life threatening. The tick carries *R. rickettsii* bacteria. The wood tick is the principal carrier in the western states whereas the dog tick and Lone-Star tick predominate in the eastern and southern parts of the United States. Rabbits and other small animals also carry this tick. Incidence is high in children under 15 years. Usually it is seasonal, May through September, except in the southern states, where it is all year. It takes at least 18 hours for a tick to bite and transmit their infection to a person—so discovering them as soon as possible is important. Untreated, this may be fatal in some cases.

PRECAUTIONS: Tick bites are painless and you will not feel them attach to you, so do the following:

1. Wear light-colored clothing so you can spot the dark brown tick.
2. Tuck your pant cuffs into your socks.
3. Examine yourself or your children several times.
4. Ticks like warm, moist parts of the body or folds of skin—check all of these areas carefully. They also like hair—so check scalp, under arms, and in the genital area as well.
5. Pets should be examined thoroughly when they get home.

SIGNS, SYMPTOMS & INDICATORS:

1. Onset is ABRUPT.
2. Severe headache.
3. Chills.
4. Fever reaching 103–104 degrees F. It may remain high for as long as 15 to 20 days in severe cases.
5. Muscular pains.
6. Weakness.
7. Nausea/vomiting.
8. Skin rash occurs on the fourth day of the fever—usually on the wrists, ankles, palms, soles, and forearms. It then moves rapidly to the neck, face, armpits, buttocks, and finally, the trunk of the body.
9. Restlessness.
10. Insomnia.
11. Delirium (fever).
12. Coma.
13. Pneumonia.
14. Heart attack.

TREATMENT:

EMERGENCY MEDICAL RESPONSE:

1. Remove the tick with tweezers by pulling straight out of the skin. Do not worry if the head of the tick remains. It is more important to remove the body, which harbors the bacteria. See your physician right away.
2. Paint area with a disinfectant.
3. Save the tick so it can be identified. Do NOT handle the tick with your fingers! Wear rubber or latex gloves.

HOMEOPATHIC: Consult a homeopath for follow-up treatment.

AFTER REMOVING THE TICK:

1. **Rhus Toxicodendron 30C**, one dose an hour. Up to six doses.
2. **Pyrogenium 30C** if bite site becomes septic (blood poisoning). See MD and homeopath right away.
3. **Ledum 30C**, one dose every hour IF bite site is COLD to your touch.

NOTES _____

_____

_____

_____

_____

★SCORPION STING★

DEFINITION: Only 4% of scorpion stings are fatal. Some species of scorpion in Arizona are deadly. Their sting is systemic and can bring about circulatory collapse. There is antivenin treatment available, but it has side effects.

SIGNS, SYMPTOMS & INDICATORS:

1. Localized swelling (not so for bark scorpion—which is deadly—where there is NO swelling at the sting site).
2. Pain.
3. Discoloration of the skin.
4. Severe muscle contractions, cramping.
5. Excessive drooling.
6. Hypertension—high blood pressure.
7. Convulsions.
8. Cardiac failure.

TREATMENT:

EMERGENCY MEDICAL RESPONSE:
1. If in Arizona, where the deadly scorpions are located, call 911 immediately.
2. Epinephrine shot (EpiPen or EpiPen Jr., if anaphylactic reaction) should be given if available (some people with severe allergy reactions or asthma carry the "Eppie" shot with them—ask if they have it—and have them administer it to themselves).
3. Wash the area with soap and water.
4. Cold pack or ice (place a cloth between ice and skin first).
5. Perform CPR if necessary.
6. If they go into shock, treat for shock. (See Shock, page 140.)

HOMEOPATHIC: Consult a homeopath for follow-up treatment.
1. **Lachesis 30C** , one dose every 15 minutes. Up to six doses.
2. **Androctonus 30C**, one dose every 15 minutes. Up to six doses. Acts like antivenin, but without the side effects. Potentized scorpion.
3. **Hypericum 30C**, one dose every 15 minutes. Up to six doses.
4. **Ledum 30C**, one dose every 15 minutes. Up to six doses.

NOTES _____

_____

_____

★SCRAPED SKIN★
(Abrasion)
See: Soft Tissue Injuries

DEFINITION: The skin is scraped off; blood oozes from the area. Possible pain, swelling, and bruising.

SIGNS, SYMPTOMS & INDICATORS:

1. Bleeding.
2. Pain.
3. Swelling.
4. Bruising

TREATMENT:

EMERGENCY MEDICAL RESPONSE:
1. Wash off and apply a clean, dry, sterile dressing.

IF A SERIOUS WOUND:
1. Control bleeding—place a sterile, dry dressing over the wound and apply direct pressure. If that does not work, apply indirect pressure on either the brachial or femoral artery. (See Bleeding, page 38.)
2. Prevent further contamination of the injury site.
3. Immobilize the affected part.
4. Use roller bandage to keep dressing in place. Then splint to hold in place.

HOMEOPATHIC:
1. Clean injury with diluted **Calendula** or **Hypericum** tincture 1:10 (1 teaspoon in a quart of water). Rinse the area well. Bandage with a dry sterile dressing.
2. Depending upon the severity of the abrasion, take **Arnica Montana 30C** as needed for localized swelling of the region. No more than six doses, an hour apart.

NOTES _____

_____

_____

_____

_____

★SHOCK★

See: Fainting

DEFINITION: Failure of the circulatory system to perfuse the cells/organs with oxygen and nutrients and to take out carbon dioxide and other waste products. Reasons for shock are pump (heart) failure (the heart beats too slow, too fast, or has lost too much muscle to squeeze hard enough due to chronic disease), vessel failure where arteries dilate and are unable to constrict, blood loss, hypovolemia where there is bleeding or fluid loss, and respiratory failure as in the case of emphysema, allergic reaction, asthma, and so forth.

SIGNS, SYMPTOMS & INDICATORS:

1. Rise in pulse—it gets thready and fast.
2. Restless and anxious—a feeling of impending doom.
3. Poor urinary output—they do not pee very much at all.
4. Falling blood pressure—one of the last signs, indicating worsening of the shock.
5. Sweaty.
6. Skin is cool and clammy feeling.
7. Skin pale and ashen.
8. Shortness of breath—air hunger.
9. Nausea and vomiting.
10. Breathing is shallow, rapid, irregular, gasping, or labored.
11. Eyes lose their luster and are black and dull looking; pupils are dilated.
12. Decreased level of consciousness.
13. Decreased capillary refill (see page 11). The fingernail beds should turn pink in 2 seconds—any longer indicates that they are going into shock.
14. Thirsty; water is requested (do not provide any).

TREATMENT:

EMERGENCY MEDICAL RESPONSE:
1. Secure the airway. Perform CPR if necessary.
2. Control the bleeding with direct pressure on the wound or use indirect pressure points—radial/femoral artery. As a LAST resort, use a tourniquet. (See Bleeding, page 38.)
3. Elevate extremities but keep them lying down on their back.
4. Splint fractures. The pain of a broken limb can keep them in shock or deepen their shock. Splinting relieves a lot of pain, therefore reducing shock.

5. Avoid rough handling—be gentle with the person.
6. Prevent loss of body heat. Place a blanket over and possibly under them (if they are lying on the ground).
7. No food or drink. They can lose consciousness and then vomit, creating an airway blockage.

HOMEOPATHIC:
NOTE: See individual types of shock below for remedy suggestions. Consult a homeopath for follow-up treatment.

TYPES OF SHOCK:

SEE: Allergic (Anaphylactic) Shock.
SEE: Fainting (Psychogenic) Shock.

Cardiogenic Shock

DEFINITION: Pump failure—the heart fails to pump adequately. It may be due to an overdose of prescription medication drugs. Or the heart can pump too fast or too slow. Congestive heart failure, where edema builds up in the body, is an example of this.

TREATMENT:

EMERGENCY MEDICAL RESPONSE: See Shock, page 140.

HOMEOPATHIC:
1. **Cactus Grandiflorus 30C**, one dose every 10 minutes. Up to six doses.
2. **Aconitum Napellus 30C**, one dose every 10 minutes for anxiety or panic—they think they are going to die. Up to six doses.
3. **Digitalis 30C**, one dose every 10 minutes. Up to six doses.

Hypovolemic Shock

DEFINITION: Failure of an organ, system or blood loss—low volume of blood in the body. It can be a cut artery, the liver bleeding, a six-day flu with vomiting/diarrhea, or a bleeding ulcer, for example. Caused by bleeding and/or dehydration.

TREATMENT:

EMERGENCY MEDICAL RESPONSE: See Shock, page 140.

HOMEOPATHIC:
1. **Arnica Montana 30C**, every 15 minutes until stable or up to six doses, if there is loss of blood.
2. **China 30C**, every 15 minutes if loss of fluids is via diarrhea, vomiting, or blood loss. Up to six doses.

Metabolic Shock

DEFINITION: Loss of fluids from the body. Caused by vomiting, diarrhea, hemorrhaging/blood loss, or too much urination, as seen in some types of flu or a severe case of food poisoning. (See Food Poisoning, page 92.)

TREATMENT:

EMERGENCY MEDICAL RESPONSE: See Shock, page 140.

HOMEOPATHIC:
1. **Ipecac 30C**, one dose every 15 minutes to halt vomiting. Up to six doses.
2. **China 30C**, one dose every 15 minutes for weakness and decreased levels of consciousness. Up to six doses.
3. **Veratrum Album 30C**, one dose every 15 minutes for acute diarrhea where electrolytes are unstable. Up to six doses.

Neurogenic Shock

DEFINITION: The nerves lose control over the arteries' ability to contract when there is trauma to the spinal cord. Below the spinal column injury, the arteries become fully dilated (blood pools below the injury site). You have vessel failure. Caused by disruption of the central nervous system (brain and/or spinal cord).

TREATMENT:

EMERGENCY MEDICAL RESPONSE: See Shock, page 140.

HOMEOPATHIC:
1. **Hypericum 30C**, one dose every 15 minutes. Up to six doses.
2. **Arsenicum Album 30C**, every 15 minutes for person who is very cold but conscious. Up to six doses.
3. **Carbo Vegetabilis 30C**, every 15 minutes for person who has moist skin, clammy with hot perspiration. Up to six doses.
4. **Arnica Montana 30C**, every 15 minutes for person who has a hot head and cold body. Up to six doses.
5. **Aconitum Napellus 30C**, every 15 minutes for person who has hot hands but feet are cold. Up to six doses.
6. **Veratrum Album 30C**, every 15 minutes for person who is cold and clammy all over. Up to six doses.

Respiratory Shock

DEFINITION: Insufficient oxygen in the blood; for example, asthma, emphysema, or pneumonia. It can also be a foreign object in the mouth blocking the airway.

TREATMENT:

EMERGENCY MEDICAL RESPONSE: See Shock, page 140.

HOMEOPATHIC:
1. **Carbo Vegetabilis 30C**, one dose every 15 minutes. Up to six doses.
2. If the person has stopped breathing, perform CPR and give **Opium 30C**, one dose every 15 minutes (one drop on underside of wrist and rub in). Up to six doses.

Septic Shock

DEFINITION: A non-vascular type of shock. Caused by a bacterial infection with high fever and blood poisoning. This is seen after surgery or complications from a very serious illness. Long-lasting and severe infection or dead tissues are involved. It can be an acute or chronic disease. It affects the arteries' ability to constrict. Hypovolemic as well as neurogenic shock will set in.

TREATMENT:

EMERGENCY MEDICAL RESPONSE: See Shock, page 140.

HOMEOPATHIC:
1. **Pyrogenium 30C**, one dose every 15 minutes. Up to six doses.
2. **Baptisia Tinctoria 30C**, one dose every 15 minutes. Up to six doses.

NOTES

★SHORTNESS OF BREATH★
(Dyspnea)

DEFINITION: Difficult or labored breathing or shortness of breath. There are many reasons; those listed below are the most life threatening.

LUNG DISORDERS—Types of Situations:

1. Pulmonary blood vessels are separated from the alveoli (where the exchange of oxygen with carbon dioxide takes place in our lungs) by fluid and/or infection.
2. Damaged alveoli cannot transport gases (oxygen, carbon dioxide) properly across their walls.
3. Spasms or mucus block the air passages in the lungs.
4. Lungs cannot expand because the pleural space is filled with air.

CAUSES OF DYSPNEA:

1. Infections of the upper or lower airways.
2. Acute pulmonary edema.
3. Chronic obstructive pulmonary diseases, such as chronic emphysema, bronchitis, or asthma.
4. Spontaneous pneumothorax.
5. Allergic reactions and asthma.
6. Mechanical obstruction of the airway (a child choking on a toy).
7. Pulmonary embolism.
8. Hyperventilation.
9. Croup.
10. Epiglottitis—the upper airway is involved. The flap or epiglottis is swollen two to three times its normal size. This flap protects the opening to the larynx.

SEE: Asthma, Croup, Emphysema, Epiglottitis, and Hyperventilation.

NOTES _____

_____

_____

_____

_____

★SNAKE BITES—POISONOUS★

DEFINITION: "Envenomation" (poison injected by a snake into a person's bloodstream) does not occur in 27% of all bites, and 37% involve only minimal envenomation. **If you do not have symptoms within an hour of the snake bite, you did not get the venom at all.** Poisonous snakes may have expended their venom on another animal, or they may bite at an angle, or your clothing may protect you from receiving a full dose. See Coral Snake, page 59, if bitten by one. The information here refers to the Pit Viper family, such as rattlesnakes, copperheads, and cottonmouths.

SIGNS, SYMPTOMS & INDICATORS:

1. Severe burning at the bite site.
2. Followed quickly by swelling and discoloration of the skin. The above signs occur within 5 to 10 minutes of the bite and spread slowly over the next 36 hours.
3. Skin will take on a bruising color—a bluish/reddish/purple discoloration.
4. Weakness.
5. Sweating.
6. Fainting from the fear of being bitten by the snake, in some instances, shortly after the bite. If the person faints HOURS afterward, this is a sign of poisoning. (See Fainting, page 91.)
7. Treat for shock. (See Shock, page 140.)
8. Localized destruction of the skin around the bite area.
9. Vomiting caused by anxiety, not by the toxin.

TREATMENT:

EMERGENCY MEDICAL RESPONSE:
1. Keep the person quiet and calmly reassure them.
2. Clean gently with soap and water or a mild antiseptic around the bite site.
3. Be alert for vomiting due to an anxiety reaction.
4. Give no fluids or food by mouth, especially alcohol.
6. Immobilize the area with a splint. Keep extremity BELOW the level of the heart.
7. Treat for shock.
8. If the snake has been killed, show it to 911 responders—they will bring it with them for identification purposes. It may be very important for antivenin purposes. Do NOT try to capture the snake—you may be bitten! Try to remember the color pattern/variation and unexaggerated size.

9. Notify 911 that it is a snake bite emergency and try to describe the snake to them in detail, if possible.

HOMEOPATHIC:
1. **Lachesis 30C**, one dose as soon after the bite as possible. Give every 15 minutes. Up to six doses.
2. **Crotalus Horridus 30C**, one dose every 15 minutes. Up to six doses.
3. **Pyrogenium 30C**, after the person is stabilized and 48 hours after bite. This prevents tissue destruction and protects against a potential septic condition. Consult a homeopath before taking this remedy.

NOTES _____

_____

_____

_____

_____

★SOFT TISSUE INJURIES★

See: Bruise, Cut, Puncture Wound, or Scraped Skin

Avulsion

DEFINITION: A piece of skin is torn completely loose and is left hanging as a flap. NOTE: It can also be or mean an amputation.

TREATMENT:

EMERGENCY MEDICAL RESPONSE:

1. Clean off the area as best you can—especially at an accident site, and lay the flap of skin back over the area and cover it with a clean, dry, sterile dressing.
2. If this is a partial amputation, clean off the best you can and wrap in a dry sterile dressing.
3. If a full amputation, sprinkle a few drops of water into a ziplock bag before adding the amputated part, which is wrapped in a dry sterile dressing. This keeps it moist. Keep in a cool place for transport. Do NOT put ice directly on the amputated part or lay it directly on top of ice. Do NOT put water or any other liquid in the bag with the amputated part. Apply direct or indirect pressure to slow or halt the bleeding.

HOMEOPATHIC:

1. Clean and flush well under and over the flap with Tincture of **Calendula** or **Hypericum**, 1:10 (1 teaspoon per quart of water). Bandage afterward with a dry sterile dressing.
2. **Arnica Montana 30C**, one dose every 15 minutes as needed for localized swelling of the region. Up to six doses.
3. If this is an amputation, **Arnica Montana 30C**, one dose every 15 minutes. Up to six doses. Consult a homeopath as soon as possible for follow-up treatment.
4. **China 30C**, one dose every 15 minutes, especially if blood loss is severe or life threatening and the person is shocky after the amputation. Up to six doses.
5. **Ignatia Amara 30C**, one dose every 15 minutes, if hysterical over the amputation. Up to six doses.
6. **Hypericum 30C**, one dose for phantom limb pain due to the amputation. It will have a nerve-like radiating pain. Consult a homeopath before taking this remedy.

Hematoma

DEFINITION: A pool of blood somewhere in the body beneath the skin or organ that is caused by a damaged large blood vessel (as opposed to blunt trauma where there is no large blood vessel involved). This may occur with serious car accidents, as an example.

SIGNS, SYMPTOMS & INDICATORS:

1. Pain at the site of the injury.
2. Swelling beneath the skin.
3. Bruising.
4. The above may be very mild to quite extensive.

TREATMENT:

EMERGENCY MEDICAL RESPONSE:
1. Watch for shock and treat. (See Hypovolemic Shock, page 141.)
2. Apply ice or a cold pack to the local site of the bruise with firm compression over the area with your hand.
3. If severe, splint the area to immobilize.
4. Elevate the affected part.

HOMEOPATHIC: Consult a homeopath for follow-up treatment.
1. **Arnica Montana 30C**, one dose every 15 minutes. Up to six doses.
2. If severe injury, **Arnica Montana 30C**, one dose every 15 minutes. Up to six doses. Follow with **Bellis Perennis 30C** if there are any remaining symptoms, one dose a day for 4 days.

IF AN EYE INJURY:
3. **Aconitum Napellus 30C**, one dose every 15 minutes. Up to six doses.
4. **Symphytum 30C**, one dose every 15 minutes. Up to six doses.

NOTES _____

_____

_____

_____

_____

★SPINAL INJURIES★

DEFINITION: The spinal cord is enclosed by vertebrae and discs, which protect it. Any kind of a fall or blow can cause one of these vertebrae to fracture or compress and put pressure on the spinal cord itself, or the nerves that run from it, known as the peripheral nerves. It is better to assume spinal injury than to ignore it. There is often no visible indicator of spinal damage, especially if the person is unconscious. To move a person can mean paralysis for life. Move them only if they are in life-threatening danger.

TREATMENT:

EMERGENCY MEDICAL RESPONSE:
1. Call 911 as soon as possible.
2. Do NOT move the person. Perform an examination. See Chapter 2, Primary and Secondary Survey, for step-by-step examination procedures (pages 9–12). Check for bruising, swelling at the injury site, deformity along the spinal column, irregularity of the vertebrae (also known as 'step-outs'), or any point of tenderness along it. Also check hands, arms, feet, and legs for any loss or decrease of sensation in them. Watch for shock to set in and treat if necessary. (See Shock, page 140.)
3. Do NOT elevate the head or neck area. If possible, a second person should firmly hold the person's head in a neutral, in-line position to keep the neck from being moved at all until 911 help can arrive.
4. Keep the entire body from moving. If you have to move the person, use a log roll (see page 16).
5. If the injured person is not breathing, use a special technique known as a 'modified jaw thrust' which moves the jaw up and outward but does NOT move the neck. (See page 18 for illustration of modified jaw thrust.) Perform CPR.
6. Question the person or witnesses about the nature of the accident.
7. Ask the person where they feel tingling, weakness, or numbness.
8. Ask the injured person to wriggle their fingers and toes. Ask them to hold out their hands (if possible) and try to resist as you **gently** push down on them. Then, place your hands beneath their palms and ask them to try to resist as you **gently** push upward—see if there is strength in the person's response. Ask them to squeeze your fingers with their hands. If they cannot do one of these, this indicates a possible spinal injury. Touch the inside and outside of their leg and ask them which leg you are touching, and which side of their leg is being touched. If they do not answer correctly, this also confirms spinal cord injury.

9. If any of the above symptoms occur, assume there IS a spinal injury and do NOT move the person until 911 help arrives.

10. If there is serious bleeding, apply a compress with direct pressure on it until help arrives. If that does not halt the bleeding, apply pressure on either the brachial or femoral artery site. (See Bleeding, page 38.)

HOMEOPATHY:

1. **Arnica Montana 30C**, every 15 minutes. This will reduce tissue swelling as well as address possible shock symptoms. Up to six doses. Consult with a homeopath as soon as possible so they can prescribe higher potency or another more suitable remedy.

2. **Hypericum 30C**. Consult a homeopath as soon as possible, as it is crucial to give the remedy right away when there are spinal cord/paralysis injuries.

NOTES _____

_____

_____

_____

_____

★SPRAIN★

DEFINITION: An injury where a person's ligaments are stretched or torn. Ligaments are bands of fibrous tissue that connect bone to bone. They support and strengthen the joint.

SIGNS, SYMPTOMS & INDICATORS:

1. Tenderness.
2. Swelling.
3. Inability to use the limb.

TREATMENT:

EMERGENCY MEDICAL RESPONSE:

1. If a ligament is sprained between two joints, splint above and below the joint.
2. If the sprain is at a joint, splint above and below it.
3. Keep weight off of it.
4. **RICE** therapy: Rest, Ice, Compression and Elevation.
   a. Rest. First 1 or 2 days allow the area to rest completely. Then exercise the joint gently without putting weight on it. You may need physical therapy, depending upon the severity. See your doctor for further instructions first.
   b. Ice pack or bag of frozen vegetables (place a towel between the ice bag and the skin) and either hold it on or use an elastic bandage. Continue ice treatment for 20 minutes at 1 or 2 hour intervals if awake. After 24 hours, switch to heat and soak joint in hot (not burning) water for 15 minutes at a time, every 2 hours if possible.
   c. Compression. Use an elastic bandage around the injured area.
   d. Elevate the extremity. Do this when you sleep; also place a small pillow beneath the area so the excess fluid can drain out of the area instead of collecting there overnight.

HOMEOPATHIC:

1. **Ruta Graveolens 30C**, one dose every 15 minutes, if it is WORSE with continued movement. Up to six doses.
2. **Rhus Toxicodendron 30C**, one dose every 15 minutes, if it is BETTER with movement. Up to six doses.

3. **Bellis Perennis 30C**, one dose every 15 minutes, if neither of the above remedies are working
4. **Symphytum 30C** helps to heal ligaments sooner and faster. Consult a homeopath about this first.

NOTES _____

_____

_____

_____

_____

_____

_____

★STRAIN★

DEFINITION: Usually called a muscle pull, it is a stretch or tearing of muscle. There is no ligament or joint damage. If there is, it becomes a sprain—see below for more information.

SIGNS, SYMPTOMS & INDICATORS:

1. Tenderness.
2. Swelling.
3. Inability to use the limb.

TREATMENT:

EMERGENCY MEDICAL RESPONSE:

1. If a muscle is strained between two joints, splint above and below the joint.
2. If a strain occurs at a joint, splint above and below it.
3. Keep your weight off of it.
4. **RICE** therapy: Rest, Ice, Compression and Elevation.
   a. Rest. First 1 or 2 days allow the area to rest completely. Then exercise the joint gently without putting weight on it. You may need physical therapy, depending upon the severity. See your doctor for further instructions first.
   b. Ice pack or a bag of frozen vegetables (place a towel between the ice bag and the skin) and either hold it on or use an elastic bandage. Continue ice treatment for 20 minutes at 1 or 2 hour intervals if awake. After 24 hours, switch to heat and soak the joint in hot (not burning) water for 15 minutes at a time, every 2 hours if possible.
   c. Compression. Use an elastic bandage around the injured area.
   d. Elevate the extremity. Do this when you sleep; also place a small pillow beneath the area so the excess fluid can drain out of the area instead of collecting there overnight.

HOMEOPATHIC:

1. **Ruta Graveolens 30C**, one dose every 15 minutes, if it is WORSE with continued movement. Up to six doses.
2. **Rhus Toxicodendron 30C**, one dose every 15 minutes, if it is BETTER with movement. Up to six doses.

3. **Bellis Perennis 30C**, one dose every 15 minutes, if neither of the above remedies are working.
4. **Symphytum 30C** helps to heal ligaments sooner and faster. Consult a homeopath about this first.

NOTES _____

_____

_____

_____

_____

_____

★STROKE★

DEFINITION: Known as a CVA or cerebrovascular accident, it occurs when the blood flow to the brain is interrupted long enough to damage some part of the brain. The brain needs a continuous flow of oxygen to function. If this is interrupted for more than 4 to 5 minutes, damage occurs. Each part of our brain is responsible for certain functions in our body.

If a stroke is suffered, for example, in the right side of the brain, it will cause problems and paralysis on the left side of the body. If this happens, the speech center can become affected and the ability to speak may be lost. Strokes can be fatal.

There are many types of strokes: Thrombosis is the most common type of stroke (the artery walls are narrowed and a clot can form inside it, suddenly and completely cutting off the blood flow). Arterial rupture occurs when an artery in the brain bursts and bleeds out into the brain itself. The artery, if it spasms to shut down the blood flow to stop the hemorrhage, further shuts off circulation to that part of the brain and more damage occurs—lack of oxygen, which kills more brain cells. The third type is known as an aneurysm. This happens when there is a weak and dilated or ballooning wall of a vessel in the brain. It is usually a congenital condition found at the base of the brain that has been there since birth. This is usually the cause of younger people having a stroke.

The reasons for stroke may also include high blood pressure and the bleeding may come from a weakened artery that is damaged by arteriosclerosis, or it can involve a healthy artery that is just simply having too much pressure exerted within it, and it ruptures and bleeds out. Another type of stroke is known as a cerebral embolism. A blood clot forms somewhere else—usually the left side of the heart, and it travels up into the head into one of the cerebral arteries and obstructs it. Blood clots will often form on a damaged or diseased heart valve. The embolus is not always a blood clot, either. It can be particles from a degenerated blood vessel wall that may break loose and travel as an emboli and create the same outcome in the cerebral artery.

SIGNS, SYMPTOMS & INDICATORS:

1. Numbness, tingling, or paralysis of extremities (right or left side, but sometimes both sides are involved).
2. Confusion and/or dizziness. Change in behavior or personality.
3. Slurred speech.
4. Facial drooping or slackness of facial muscles along with drooling. Loss of muscle control on one side of the body.
5. Diminished level of consciousness.

6. Seizures.
7. Incontinence (they may wet their pants).
8. Severe headache before the stroke.
9. They may have difficulty breathing, speaking, or seeing.

TREATMENT:

EMERGENCY MEDICAL RESPONSE:
1. Ask them if they are okay. If they do not or cannot respond, have someone call 911.
2. Check airway and make sure they can breathe and that they have a pulse. If they do not, begin CPR.
3. If the person is conscious and breathing, GENTLY raise their head about 6 inches above the rest of the body and make them comfortable. Place a blanket over them to keep them warm, but not hot.
4. Calm them and reassure them until medical help arrives.

HOMEOPATHIC: Consult a homeopath IMMEDIATELY after making the 911 call for follow-up treatment.
1. **Arnica Montana 30C**, every 15 minutes until help arrives. Up to six doses.
2. Contact your homeopath. The sooner the injured person can get the appropriate remedy, the less damage will be created by the stroke.

    TIME IS OF THE ESSENCE!

NOTES   _____

_____

_____

_____

_____

★TICK BITES★

See: Lyme Disease and Rocky Mountain Spotted Fever

DEFINITION: There are two types of disease being spread, Lyme disease and Rocky Mountain Spotted Fever. Both are covered here. Lyme disease, after AIDS, is the second most contagious and infectious disease in the United States! It originally began in Connecticut, but is now reported in 43 other states.

SEE: Page 120 for Lyme Disease.
SEE: Page 136 for Rocky Mountain Spotted Fever.

NOTES _____

_____

_____

_____

_____

Chapter 4

HOMEOPATHIC MATERIA MEDICA A–Z

A Materia Medica (medical materials) is simply a compilation of symptoms that, if a healthy person took this remedy, would cause this specific set of symptoms in them. To a homeopath it is a listing of symptoms that have been caused by the remedy listed.

The easiest way to use the Materia Medica is to match, as closely as possible, the injured person's symptoms to the remedy. **If there are three or more symptom 'matches' then use the remedy.** If there is one or two, do not. Go on to the next suggested remedy and look it up and see if you get a closer agreement on symptom matches.

If there is no symptom match (three or more) do NOT give them a homeopathic remedy. Do what you can as outlined in the Emergency Medical Response section and wait for 911 medical responders to arrive.

ACONITUM NAPELLUS
(Aconite)

1. This remedy has been used for SHOCK of any kind. It covers 90% of all shock symptoms. Used for flu, colds, convulsions, all kinds of eye injuries, Hyphema, shortness of breath, paralysis, among others.
2. Anxiety or fear following the incident/accident.
3. Very thirsty; usually for cool or cold drinks.
4. Bitter taste in mouth.
5. Urine retention after accident/trauma—cannot pee.
6. Fears of dying.
7. Restlessness.
8. Flushed, sweaty face; one cheek red/the other white.
9. Panicky or anxiety reaction.
10. All symptoms come on after the fright/trauma/accident.
11. For foreign objects in one's eye.
12. Sudden blindness after experiencing trauma/shock.
13. Angina or acute myocardial infarction (heart attack) with numbness into the left arm.
14. Sudden heat and chills.
15. Pupils constricted—black portions of eyes are pinpoints. Eyes red and inflamed, deep redness of the vessels, and intolerable pain.
16. Profuse lachrymation (tears or tearing from the eyes).
17. Pupil(s) is DILATED (opened wide—looks black and huge).
18. Black spots and mist before the eyes, disturbed by 'flickering' or vision as if through a veil, difficult to distinguish faces.
19. Eyelids feel dry, hard, heavy, and sensitive to air.
20. Cannot bear sunlight or reflection of snow—it causes specks, sparks and scintillations to dance before the eyes.
21. 'Drawing' (pulling) sensation in the eyelids with drowsiness.
22. Cold hands and feet.
23. Symptoms are WORSE while in warm room, in the evening and night, lying on the injured side, from music playing, from being exposed to cigarette smoke or to cold/dry wind or draft, from being scared to death (frightened), while sweating, chilled by a cold wind, in dry weather, from expressing or feeling violent emotions, or sleeping out in sunlight.
24. Symptoms are BETTER in open air, from rest, or from warm sweat.

NOTES _____

_____

_____

AGARICUS MUSCARIUS
(Toad Stool—Bug Agaric)

1. This remedy has been used in chilblains, seizure disorders, and other pathologies. It is a major frostnip and frostbite remedy.
2. Pains are accompanied by sensation of cold, numbness, and tingling of affected part.
3. Burning, itching, redness, and swelling.
4. Swollen veins with cold skin.
5. Tearing, contractive pain in muscles.
6. Itching of toes and feet as if frozen.
7. Face muscles feel stiff, may be twitching.
8. Lancing, tearing pain in cheeks; feels like splinters.
9. Nerves feel as if cold needles ran through them or sharp ice touched them. Sensation of cold or hot needles to frozen skin.
10. Face colored blue and puffy looking.
11. Itching area that changes places and moves once it is scratched.
12. Limbs stiff all over.
13. Yawning a great deal.
14. Symptoms are WORSE from being out in open cold or freezing air, from touch, in the sun, and after alcohol consumption.
15. Symptoms are BETTER from moving about slowly.

SEE: **Laurocerasus**, **Petroleum** for frostnip/frostbite conditions.

NOTES _____

_____

_____

_____

_____

ALLIUM CEPA

(Red Onion)

1. This remedy is useful in upper respiratory infections, colds, coughs, otitis media, pertussis, and allergies, among others.
2. Acrid nasal discharge from the nose, but discharge from eyes is bland.
3. Tearing pain in the larynx while coughing.
4. Sensation as if a thread between neck and head.
5. Hoarseness.
6. Sensation as if throat is split or torn.
7. Pain in throat extending to the ear when coughing.
8. Tickling in larynx.
9. Sensation of lump in throat.
10. Symptoms are WORSE in a warm room, damp weather, in the evening, resting, or when lying down.
11. Symptoms are BETTER in open air, a cooler room (air conditioning), bathing, or from moving around.

NOTES _____

_____

_____

_____

_____

ANDROCTONUS AMURREUXI
(Scorpion)

1. This remedy has been used for salivation, strabismus, and tetanus. In an emergency, if no other homeopathic remedy worked on a scorpion bite, this should be thought of—providing the symptoms fit.
2. Anxiety, panic, changeable mood (can be friendly one moment and angry, combative the next), uncontrollable temper. Can be dreamy-appearing, depressed, and detached from what is going on to them or around them.
3. Lack of concentration, difficulty with any mental task. Mind goes 'blank.' Forgetful. Absent-minded.
4. Skin is pale looking or red, sore, itching, and with eruptions.
5. Soles of feet and palms of hands around the veins become red, sore, painful, and itching.
6. Anxiety felt in stomach. Nausea, very thirsty. Vomiting with only bile coming up. Sharp pains around the belly button.
7. Pain in tongue, as if hot needles. Tongue sore, enlarged, and tingling or numbness.
8. Chill in upper back and shoulder area.
9. Perspiration is profuse and does not alleviate symptoms.
10. Diarrhea is explosive, smells like fish.
11. Symptoms are WORSE at 9 pm, after drinking orange juice, from motion, standing or sitting up, or from being touched.
12. Symptoms are BETTER after midnight, consuming hot drinks, lying down, or taking a hot bath.

NOTES _____

_____

_____

_____

_____

ANTIMONIUM TARTARICUM
(Tartar Emetic)

1. This remedy has been used for bronchitis, chronic obstructive pulmonary disease, congestive heart failure, cyanosis, pneumonia, respiratory infections, croup, and sepsis, among others.
2. Difficult breathing, relieved by coughing up mucus, or expectoration of fluid in lungs.
3. Wet cough but person is not able to cough mucus up.
4. Rattling sound in chest and throat region.
5. Uses accessory muscles to breathe (often seen in emphysema).
6. Fluid in the lungs and suffocation from it.
7. Cyanosis (blueness) around lips, eyes, finger or toenail beds or other parts of the body due to respiratory condition and being unable to breathe or get enough oxygen into the body.
8. Nausea and vomiting with a cough.
9. May be irritable and peevish during the trauma.
10. Does not want to be touched by anyone.
11. Increasingly weak and sweaty; becomes drowsy and relaxed with lack of reaction.
12. Great accumulation of mucus in chest, rattling sounds are heard; breathing is impeded and heart action is very labored as a result.
13. Infants nursing at the nipple will let go and cry, as if out of breath.
14. Pale, covered with a cold sweat, incessant quivering of the chin and lower jaw.
15. Thirst for cold water—little and often.
16. Nostrils are widely flared (to get maximum amount of oxygen into their body).
17. Coarse, loose, rattling cough, chest seems full of mucus, yet less and less raised with each breath.
18. Symptoms are WORSE from warmth, being in a warm room, wrapped in a blanket, in warm weather, from being angry, in the morning, becoming overheated, from cold dampness, sitting down, or from drinking milk.
19. Symptoms are BETTER from sitting erect, from belching and expectoration of mucus, from motion, vomiting, belching, and lying on their right side.

NOTES _____

_____

_____

_____

APIS MELLIFICA
(Honeybee)

1. This remedy has been used for anaphylactic (allergic) reaction, swelling, sore throat disorders, allergic shock, asthma, injuries that involve swelling, puncture wounds, stroke, and effects of surgery, among others.
2. Swelling of the skin, with redness of skin, heat, and itching.
3. The injured area is worse from heat being applied to it.
4. Stinging pains.
5. For allergic/anaphylaxis reaction.
6. Edema (swelling) beneath the skin, making the skin feel very tight with a constricted sensation to it.
7. Swelling of the throat and uvula.
8. Eyes—swelling of the conjuctiva, which are red, burning, and better with application of cold to the area.
9. Shortness of breath, hurried and difficult breathing. Feels as if they cannot draw another breath into their body.
10. Whole body may puff or swell up after a bite of some kind.
11. Symptoms are WORSE from heat in any form (cloth applied, temperature, or weather), from being touched, pressure applied to injured area, late in the afternoon, after sleeping, and being kept in a closed, heated room.
12. Symptoms are BETTER when they are in open air or near an open window, uncovering and taking a cold bath or shower.

SEE: **Carbolicum Acidum.**

NOTES _____

_____

_____

_____

_____

ARNICA MONTANA
(Leopard's Bane)

1. This remedy has been very useful in hemorrhaging or bleeding, trauma to the soft tissue of the body—bruises, contusions, head injuries, sprains, strains, post-surgery, and broken bones, among others.
2. Everything feels too hard—the ground, the sofa, or the bed.
3. Does not want to be touched. Person will pull away or shrink from you if you reach out to touch them.
4. They say that everything is fine, that they are okay—but they're not.
5. Head is hot, body is cold.
6. Loss of sight or hearing after trauma to head.
7. Does not want to be consoled, held, or touched.
8. Useful in blunt trauma to the eye.
9. Nosebleeds while washing their face, from coughing, or from some trauma.
10. Person has a red face after suffering a stroke.
11. Restless; cannot find a position that suits them.
12. Cannot bear the least pain—extremely sensitive to the least amount of pain.
13. Whole body overly sensitive to everything.
14. Eyes—double-vision.
15. General feeling of being bruised, sore, or lame.
16. Dizziness and vertigo (everything whirls around head). Dizzy upon closing their eyes.
17. Skin is black and blue, or bruised looking.
18. Their symptoms are WORSE from being touched, being jarred, movement, resting, getting cold from dampness, rain, or high humidity, or from any blow, shock, hard physical labor, sprains, or falls.
19. Their symptoms are BETTER lying down or with their head lower than the rest of the body, or being outstretched. NOTE: If suffering a head injury, do NOT lower the head; rather, elevate it 6 inches (so long as no spinal injury is involved).

NOTES _____

_____

_____

_____

_____

ARSENICUM ALBUM

(Arsenic Trioxide)

1. This remedy has been used in asthma, anxiety attacks, panic attacks, pneumonia, food poisoning, stomach disorders, sore throat, and others.
2. Anxious, worried and tense.
3. Great anxiety along with extreme restlessness—will not sit or stand still.
4. Fear of dying.
5. Chilly and is worse from being damp, cold, or in a draught of wind.
6. Always better with heat in any form (a blanket wrapped snugly around them, a hot drink, or being near a warm fire, etc.).
7. Anxious about the other members of their family—not themselves.
8. Burning pain in esophagus and stomach. Will want to sip cold/cool water repeatedly.
9. Craving cold drinks—but may be vomited back up immediately afterward.
10. Diarrhea that is watery, acrid, and very smelly.
11. Cannot bear the sight or smell of food.
12. Anxiety in the pit of the stomach. Burning pains. Craves coffee.
13. Long belches. Vomiting of blood, bile, green mucus, or brown-black mucus mixed with blood.
14. Stomach feels irritable, raw, as if torn.
15. Everything swallowed seems to lodge in the esophagus, which seems closed and feels as if nothing will pass beyond that point.
16. Rectum burns and has pressure in it.
17. Symptoms are WORSE from wet weather, cold dampness or cold air (air conditioning), ice, cold drinks, or cold food.
18. Symptoms are BETTER from hot, dry applications, motion or walking about (if possible), from having company, heat, warm drinks/ food, or a warm wrap around them or a blanket.

NOTES _____

_____

_____

_____

_____

BAPTISIA TINCTORIA
(Wild Indigo)

1. This remedy is used in flu symptoms, pharyngitis, septic shock, and septic conditions, among others.
2. Rapid onset of a septic fever condition—within hours the person goes from feeling well to becoming very sick.
3. Great confusion mentally. Dull. Stupor or semiconscious. Appears intoxicated or drunk.
4. Can fall asleep mid-sentence.
5. Putrid odor of mouth, stool, and perspiration—a rotten 'road kill' odor.
6. Speech is slurred and thick.
7. Bruising pains in body and muscles and no position is comfortable. The bed feels too hard.
8. Delirium. Person feels as if they are scattered all over the bed and they try to bring all these pieces together again.
9. High fever with a sudden onset.
10. Can swallow liquids only—not food. If they try to eat, they gag.
11. Cannot bear light of any kind—eyes burn and feel weak. Too painful to read anything.
12. Eyeballs feel sore and bruised.
13. Tongue feels swollen and numb, so speech is difficult. Tongue feels burnt.
14. Painless sore throat.
15. Person may appear to have drunk too much alcohol—but has not touched a drop—a besotted, drunken expression to their face.
16. Symptoms are WORSE from being out in open air, cold wind, in the Fall, during hot, humid weather, from pressure on the affected part, on walking and from walking.

SEE: **Pyrogenium**.

NOTES _____

_____

_____

_____

_____

BELLADONNA
(Deadly Nightshade)

1. This remedy has been used for arthritis, convulsions, delirium, fever-related convulsions, blunt trauma to eyes, Hyphema, otitis media, seizure disorders, and high blood pressure, among others.

2. Headache pains are aggravated by the least jarring, noise, direct or indirect light, the sun, heat, washing one's hair, stooping, or coughing. Pains are throbbing and knife-like or pulsating/pounding. May feel like brains are going to be pushed out of the skull or eye sockets.

3. Cold hands and feet, but the face is hot and red/flushed looking with pupils black and dilated.

4. Ear pain is severe, usually right-sided, and is worse at night in bed. There is a throbbing, knife-like pain in ear.

5. Emotionally explosive and they can get very angry very quickly. May strike out, try to bite you, or spit at you.

6. Hallucinations that are very vivid and real. They have a great fear of dogs.

7. Eyes are wide, staring, and brilliant/shiny looking—a vacant look to them—a "nobody is home" appearance.

8. Double vision. Objects appear double or reversed, or red in color. Pupil(s) dilated—wide open, large and black looking. Pupils immovable and generally dilated, but sometimes, also contracted (pupil tiny, black, and looks like a pinpoint in the eye) and immovable. (Immovable means the pupil(s) does not respond to various amount of light, or a flashlight being shined in them—the pupil should constrict and then dilate when light is taken away—but it does not. Pupil(s) is then said to be immovable or unresponsive to light changes.)

9. Eyes are red, staring, brilliant, and shining in appearance OR dull and turbid looking. Congestion of blood to the eye and redness of the veins.

10. Eye feels swollen and protruding. Sensation as if eye is half closed (and it is not).

11. Vision is tinted yellow—there can be like a yellow veil or coloring over everything they look at.

12. Conjunctiva is red, dry, burning with shooting pain in eye(s). Heat and burning in the eye or pressure felt as if from sand. Ache in eye and socket that extends into the head. Sensation of weight in the eyelid, which closes involuntarily. Quivering of the eyelid.

13. Mist, flame, or sparks before the eyes. Diffusion of the light of candles (or light bulb) which appear to be surrounded by a colored halo. White stars and silvery clouds before the eyes—especially when looking up at the ceiling of a room. Bright light hurts their eyes.
14. Pain causes delirium. In a child, they can cry out in their sleep.
15. Spasms, shocks, jerking and twitching of the arms and legs.
16. Symptoms come on swiftly, within minutes.
17. Skin is hot, red, and dry. There may be a 'scalded' sensation to their skin. If you put your hand near them, you can feel the heat radiating or roiling off their skin. They are like a hot stove.
18. Symptoms are WORSE from heat of the sun, if overheated, from drafts on the head, after getting a haircut or washing their hair, from light, noise, being jarred, from touch, company, motion, hanging the affected part down, lying down, looking at shining objects or being around running water. Symptoms worsen around 3 pm, although it may start around 11 am.
19. Symptoms are BETTER from a light covering, sitting semi-erect, resting in bed, standing, leaning head against something, bending, or turning the affected part.

NOTES _____

_____

_____

_____

_____

BELLIS PERENNIS
(Daisy)

1. This remedy has been used for tumors created by an old injury, sprains and strains, deep tissue injuries, dislocations, venous stasis, childbirth, blunt trauma eye injuries, Hyphema, after surgical operations, and varicose veins, among others.
2. For sore, bruised sensation (may follow Arnica if any bruises or swelling are left from a tissue-related injury).
3. For any kind of trauma, surgery, or a broken bone. Removes swelling and blood stasis from old or new injuries.
4. Sore, bruised feeling in the pelvic region, especially in an abdominal injury.
5. Bruised sore feeling to scalp.
6. Soreness of the uterine area of a woman.
7. Joint injury, muscular soreness, or joint dislocations. Sprains. There is stiffness and coldness associated with the injured region.
8. Used for hematomas (vein is torn open and blood is pooling beneath the skin to a marked degree—much more serious than just a 'bruise').
9. Postoperative pain and bruising.
10. Any kind of trauma with swelling, especially of soft tissue related injuries.
11. Can be used in old injuries that have never healed completely.
12. Eye injuries. Eye strain. Conjunctivitis with abrasion and irritating discharge.
13. Symptoms are WORSE on the left side, after a hot bath, in the warmth of the bed, before a storm, cold bathing or being in a cold wind, becoming chilled when hot, after a surgical operation, and from cold coupled with immobility.
14. Symptoms are BETTER from continued motion, cold applications, heat, eating, and pressure on the affected part.

NOTES _____

_____

_____

_____

_____

CACTUS GRANDIFLORUS
(Night Blooming Cereus Cactus)

1. This remedy is used for angina, arrhythmia, acute myocardial infarction (heart attack), valvular diseases, hemorrhage, and nosebleeds, among others.
2. Pain in heart region that is described as "gripped by an iron fist."
3. Severe, constricting, band-like pain around chest.
4. Numbness or pain moving down the left arm into the hand or fingers.
5. Oppression on the chest with a sense of suffocation—person cannot breathe, cannot draw in a breath of air.
6. Violent, severe, and constricting chest pain.
7. Pain so bad that the person cries out.
8. General aggravation at 11 am or 11 pm.
9. Choking sensation, along with constriction in the throat.
10. Cyanosis of the skin; a blue tinge around mouth or eyes, nail beds, or possibly other parts of the body.
11. Coldness in arms and legs. They will say they are 'icy' cold.
12. Heart palpitations that worsen with exertion or lying on their left side.
13. After eating, it feels like a 'lump' or weight in their stomach.
14. Symptoms get WORSE with noise, light, heat from sunlight, 11 am or 11 pm, walking, climbing stairs or up a hill, from dampness or being damp, lying down on left side, after eating a meal or missing a meal, or fasting.
15. Symptoms get BETTER by being in open air, and pressure on the top of the head (pressing with their hand or a pillow against it).

SEE: **Aconitum Napellus**

NOTES _____

_____

_____

_____

_____

CALCAREA PHOSPHORICUM
(Calcium Phosphate)

1. This remedy is known to help scoliosis, neck, and lower back pain, to heal bones that do not want to knit properly, broken bones, bone disorders, slow dentition, osteoporosis, otitis media, chronic fatigue syndrome, carpal tunnel syndrome, and arthritis, among others.
2. Pain in joints and bones.
3. Crawling and coldness on limb.
4. Stiffness and pain with cold, numb feeling in limb.
5. Delayed healing of fractures and sprains.
6. Growing pains in children.
7. Spinal column difficulties; curvature of the spine to the left.
8. Sacral (lower back) area numb and lame or weak feeling.
9. Violent pain in their back from least movement; the person may scream out in pain.
10. Buttocks, back, and limbs go to sleep and become numb feeling.
11. Symptoms are WORSE from loss of fluids (sweating, urinating, diarrhea, vomiting, bleeding), from motion, lifting or climbing, thinking about one's symptoms, changes in the weather, being exposed to dampness, cold weather, snow, or drafts.
12. Symptoms are BETTER during the summer, being warm, in a dryer atmosphere, lying down, and resting.

NOTES _____

_____

_____

_____

_____

CANTHARIS
(Spanish Fly)

1. This remedy has been used for first degree burns, sunburn, cystitis, bladder or kidney infections, or kidney disease, among others.
2. Raw, burning pain which is relieved by cold applications.
3. Pains are cutting, smarting, or burning and biting.
4. Constant urge to urinate. Straining to urinate. Blood in the urine.
5. When a person urinates, there is a scalding, cutting pain with intolerable urging. Urine may pass, drop by drop.
6. Affected or injured skin will have a burning sensation if touched.
7. Burns and scalds of the mouth and esophagus: a scalded feeling with great difficulty swallowing liquids. Throat feels painfully constricted, full of blisters. Violent spasm of the throat if touched.
8. Symptoms are WORSE after being touched, looking at bright objects, being around the sound of water, while urinating and after urinating, or drinking cold water or hot coffee.
9. Symptoms are BETTER from rubbing the affected area with a warm application, warmth and rest.

NOTES _____

_____

_____

_____

CARBO VEGETABILIS
(Vegetable Charcoal)

1. This remedy has been used for air hunger, asphyxiation, blood loss, bronchitis, labored breathing, snoring, cholera, collapsed conditions (shock), fainting, hemorrhaging, heart disease, flu, measles, laryngitis, congested lungs, mumps, hyperventilating, esophagitis, and sleep disorders, among others. It increases maximum perfusion within the body.
2. Spasmodic gagging/vomiting of mucus with respiratory problem (asthma, pneumonia, bronchitis, cardio-obstructive pulmonary disease).
3. Hyperventilation.
4. Unable to get sufficient oxygen into the body. Breath is cold.
5. For a near-drowning person.
6. Coma.
7. Asthma where skin is turning blue.
8. Skin is blue, cold, and bruised. Or may appear marble-like with veins showing beneath it.
9. Excellent for shock where person is cold and not getting sufficient oxygen.
10. Abdomen greatly extended and swollen. Better passing gas.
11. Wants fresh air immediately, will fan themselves, wants moving air around them.
12. Shortness of breath and must sit up in a chair or sit up in bed. Cold feet and legs (poor circulation).
13. Congestive heart failure with anxiety, shortness of breath, bluish color around mouth, eyes, the finger or toenail beds, bloated appearance of face or body, and they feel better fanning themselves, getting fresh air, or being on oxygen.
14. Symptoms are WORSE in the evening, at night, from getting cold, from eating fatty food, from being in warm, damp weather, or drinking wine.
15. Symptoms are BETTER by fanning themselves, getting to fresh air and cooler weather, and remaining in a cooler temperature (air conditioning).

NOTES _____

_____

_____

_____

_____

CARBOLICUM ACIDUM
(Carbolic Acid)

1. This remedy has been used for anaphylactic (allergic) reactions (to bites, stings, inhalation of an odor, food poisoning, etc.), pharyngitis, and shock, among others.
2. Face dusky red with white around the mouth and nose.
3. Cannot swallow; throat is swelling shut.
4. Allergic reaction to bee and insect stings of all kinds.
5. Shock and collapse.
6. Pulse is feeble.
7. Cannot breathe, paralysis of respiratory (lungs, diaphragm) centers.
8. Depressed breathing.
9. Swelling of face and tongue after the sting of an insect.
10. Symptoms are WORSE in a warm room, and person is sensitive to cold air/drafts.

SEE: **Apis Mellifica.**

NOTES _____

_____

_____

_____

_____

CAUSTICUM

(Potassium Hydrate)

1. This remedy is used in cases of third degree burns, creeping paralysis from trauma or accident, central nervous system disorders, allergies, arthritis, carpal tunnel syndrome, and strokes, among others.
2. Compulsively checks and then rechecks any task they are responsible for.
3. Stammering when excited or anxious.
4. Fears that bad things will happen.
5. Cough or sneezing will cause incontinence; loss of a few drops of urine.
6. Old burns that do not heal up completely. Ill effects from serious burns (second or third degree).
7. Violent itching of skin or over entire body. Especially at night. Tingling, stinging, and swelling of skin.
8. Yellowish looking skin that burns, has ulcers, corrodes, has pus or thin watery pus suppurating from injured areas. Jerking pains running through these blisters or ulcers.
9. Symptoms are WORSE in the evening 6 pm to 8 pm and from 3 am to 4 am, from physical exertion, change of weather, car motion, twilight, fine, clear weather and dry, cold air, wind, being in a draft, suffering from any extreme of temperature, drinking coffee, or cool/cold bathing.
10. Symptoms are BETTER from cold drinks, damp or wet weather, washing, warmth of the bed, and gentle motion.

NOTES _____

_____

_____

_____

_____

CHINA
(Cinchona Officinalis)

1.   This remedy has been used for shock, especially from severe blood loss or hemorrhaging, asthma, coma, food poisoning, flu, intermittent fever, strokes, tinnitus, high, debilitating fevers and diarrhea, and varicose veins, among others.
2.   Weakness and debility from loss of fluids—bleeding, sweating, urinating, vomiting, diarrhea or other vital fluids.
3.   Post-operative gas pains from abdominal surgery. There is no relief from passing it.
4.   For severe hemorrhaging situations.
5.   They will hurt other people's feelings. Apathetic. Indifferent to their situation. Depressed and taciturn. Sudden crying and tossing about. Touchy. Irritable. Supersensitive.
6.   Hard pressure on affected area relieves pain and discomfort.
7.   Coldness and much sweat. One hand is icy cold, the other is warm.
8.   Shock remedy especially when severe blood loss accompanies and complicates the condition.
9.   Gas in abdomen that is made better by person bending double. Stomach and abdomen feel cold.
10. Abdomen hard, sounds like a drum. Bloated, distended, with frequent rumblings and burping.
11. Blue color around eyes; eyes look hollow with yellow color in whites of eyes.
12. Does not want to be touched. Especially a light touch; they can tolerate a pressured type of touch much better.
13. Symptoms are WORSE from the slightest touch, being caught in a draft of air, every other day, loss of vital fluids, at night, and after eating.
14. Symptoms are BETTER from bending over double, being out in the open air or near a window that is open, and being warm.

NOTES _____

_____

_____

_____

_____

CROTALUS HORRIDUS
(Venom of the Timber Rattlesnake)

1. This remedy is useful in angina, delirium, hemorrhage (especially in poisonous snake bites), hemorrhagic fevers such as Ebola, or bacterial epidemics including the bubonic plague, yellow fever, and cholera. Acute myocardial infarction (heart attack), and septic conditions or septic shock.
2. Massive, widespread bleeding from any or all orifices of the body: eyes, ears, nose, mouth, vagina, rectum, or even from the skin itself.
3. Blood is dark colored but CANNOT clot.
4. Suspicious of those who try to help—friends, family, EMTs, or paramedics.
5. Think they are going to die; very sad and weepy; they have clouded mental perception.
6. Skin has purple and reddish areas; hemorrhaging beneath the skin. Skin of face may be sallow or yellow (jaundiced looking).
7. Lips are swollen, yellow, and have a deathlike pallor to them. May be distorted looking.
8. Unquenchable, burning thirst.
9. Spasms of the esophagus. They cannot swallow, especially liquids. A tight, constricting feeling around throat. Very thirsty.
10. Fainting if they sit upright.
11. Intolerance for tight clothing around stomach region (wants waistband of slacks/jeans opened up).
12. Sinking sensation in the stomach.
13. Moldy smell to the breath.
14. Tip of nose may appear to be blue and red.
15. Trembling feeling around the heart. Pain through left shoulder and down left arm. Pulse barely perceptible. Pain around the heart.
16. Burning in the chest, with an oppressive feeling as if someone is sitting on top of them; unable to draw in a deep breath of air.
17. Abdomen is cold as ice. Violent pains on left side of rib cage. Heat and tenderness of the abdomen—they cannot stand clothes over the area.
18. Vomiting of anything eaten. Vomiting of dark, black blood that may look like coffee grounds.
19. Nosebleed—blood is black and stringy coming out of the nostrils.
20. Symptoms are WORSE from lying on their right side, falling to sleep, drinking alcohol, being jarred, from being in damp, wet weather, cold weather, or extremely dry air, in the evening, in the morning, and after sleeping.

21. Symptoms are BETTER from rest and open air (temperature in mid-70s).

SEE: **Elaps Corallinus, Lachesis**.

NOTES _____

_____

_____

_____

_____

DIGITALIS

(Foxglove)

1. This remedy is of use in heart problems such as angina, congestive heart failure, arrhythmia, and rheumatic heart disease, among others.
2. Pulse is weak, irregular, intermittent, or abnormally slow.
3. Blueness of the eyelids (cyanosis).
4. Excessive nausea or great weakness felt in the stomach.
5. Shortness of breath; cannot take a deep breath.
6. Faintness with pallor of the skin.
7. Fear of dying from a heart attack.
8. Fear that their heart will stop beating.
9. Angina is worse after sex.
10. Heart palpitations, particularly after experiencing some traumatic grief.
11. Cannot bear to talk.
12. Swelling of the feet. Fingers go to sleep easily.
13. Coldness in the hands and feet.
14. Anxious about the future.
15. Bluish appearance to the face (cyanosis).
16. Great physical weakness from the least amount of exertion.
17. Creeping sensation over the skin.
18. Soreness to chest. Pain in chest when sitting over in a bent position. Weak sensation in chest. Pressure or tension in the chest that makes the person want to take a deep breath.
19. Symptoms are WORSE from exertion, lying on their left side, from cold drinks or food, cold weather or heat, after sex, on waking in the morning, from drinking alcohol, being raised up in bed, from being touched or pressure being put on their chest, from music, and at night.
20. Symptoms are BETTER on an empty stomach, from resting, being in cool air (or air conditioning), lying on their back, or sitting erect.

NOTES _____

_____

_____

_____

_____

ELAPS CORALLINUS
(Venom of Coral Snake)

1. This remedy is helpful in cases of angina, esophageal spasm, hemorrhage, peptic ulcers, PMS, sinusitis, as well as being bitten by a poisonous snake, among others.
2. Coldness is experienced in the stomach and chest.
3. Cravings for ice, oranges, or salads.
4. Nosebleed with BLACK appearing blood.
5. Many emotional/mental fears: of rain, they can speak but cannot be understood, of snakes, of having a stroke, of being left alone, imagines hearing someone talk (but no one is speaking), dreads being left alone. They can also be angry about themselves and do not want to be spoken to.
6. Spitting up of blood which is BLACK appearing.
7. Coldness in body is worsened by drinking cold fluids.
8. Air hunger; cannot get enough oxygen into the lungs.
9. Cold perspiration all over the body, but skin is hot and dry to touch.
10. Sensation of a sponge in the throat. Spasmodic contractions of the esophagus.
11. Breath is very foul smelling.
12. Falls forward. May faint when vomiting or stooping.
13. Face may be bloated looking, have a dull yellow color, or have red spots on it.
14. Aversion to any kind of light because it hurts their eyes. Burning in the eyelids. Bloated looking around the eyes. Letters run together when they try to read.
15. Bowels feel twisted together in a knot.
16. Great sensitivity to cold, a draft, windy conditions (including air conditioning), and rain.
17. Symptoms are WORSE when eating fruit, cold drinks, being damp or in humid weather, in rainy weather, from the approaching of a storm, being touched, and warmth of bed, or any type of exertion.
18. Symptoms are BETTER from resting; walking relieves the nosebleed and pain in abdomen/chest.

SEE: **Lachesis, Crotalus Horridus.**

NOTES _____

_____

_____

_____

FORMICA RUFA
(Red Ants)

1. This remedy has been used for arthritis, insect bites, dislocations, and spinal disorders, among others.
2. Severe pain across lower back, or pain on left side of neck when chewing.
3. Dull pain around the spleen region, flatulence, and drawing pain around the belly button.
4. Joints are stiff and are worse with motion and better if pressure (massage) is applied to the area.
5. Nettle-like rash on skin. Red, itching, and burning skin. Profuse sweat without relief.
6. Hoarseness with a sore throat.
7. Dry, sore throat with aching in forehead and constrictive, sharp, cutting pains in the chest.
8. Violent attacks of coughing with vomiting.
9. Weakness of arms and legs, hands numb, stiffness and contraction of joints with itching under armpits.
10. Heart has fluttering palpitations with an uneasy pain in that region.
11. Face, left side, feels paralyzed.
12. Headache in which bubbles feel like they are bursting out of forehead region.
13. Pain when moving eyes.
14. Symptoms are WORSE during cold weather and cold shower or bath or cold applications, damp weather, or from sitting down.
15. Symptoms are BETTER from warmth, pressure or rubbing the affected area, and after midnight.

NOTES _____

_____

_____

_____

_____

GLONOINE
(Nitroglycerin)

1. This remedy works well for heart arrhythmia, flushes, headaches, high blood pressure, menopause, sun stroke (heat stroke), and heart-valve disease, among others.
2. Sensation of pulsations (throbbing or wavelike motion) throughout the body or head.
3. Confusion with dizziness. Cannot bear any heat about their head. Throbbing headache or throbbing sensation throughout the head. A sensation of surging blood from the heart into the head.
4. Bursting and expansive sensation in the head.
5. Extreme irritability, gets excited by the slightest opposition, confusion about where they are (even if it is a familiar place).
6. Clothing seems tight to them.
7. Wants to lie down or be in the shade. Cannot stand direct sunlight at all.
8. Violent convulsions associated with cerebral congestion in the head.
9. Feels very tired; cannot work.
10. General pulsations with numbness.
11. Symptoms are WORSE from being out in the sun, exposure to the sun's rays, an open fire, tight collars, from motion, from heat/temperature, stooping, drinking any kind of stimulant (coffee/tea/soda pop), and lying down on their left side.
12. Symptoms are BETTER from being out in open air, elevating the head slightly, placing hand on head with pressure, drinking cold fluids, cold or cool applications.

SEE: **Belladonna**.

NOTES _____

_____

_____

_____

_____

HAMAMELIS
(Witch Hazel)

1. This remedy has been used for many types of venous congestion (black eye, eye injuries in general, Hyphema, bruising, gastric ulcer), such as hemorrhoids, varicose veins, hemorrhages (internal or external), for phlebitis, burns, bruises, vein inflammation and ulcers, and after operations, among others.
2. Sore pain down cervical vertebrae (the neck region). Severe pain in lower back (sacral) which extends down the legs.
3. Very sore muscles and joints.
4. Chilliness in back and hips extending down their legs.
5. Skin blue. Chilblains. Very sore feeling to the skin surface.
6. Vomiting up black blood. Nausea, which is better if they keep quiet. Trembling sensation in stomach.
7. Coughing up blood from a tickling and dry cough. Chest feels sore and constricted. Person cannot lie down due to difficult breathing and chest congestion. Worse by taking a long or deep breath. Muscles on left side of chest are dull and aching.
8. Hemorrhaging blood is slow moving and dark colored (passive bleeding)—vein or venous origin/source. Person is always sore and bruised feeling in the region that is affected.
9. Weak, cold, quick pulse with profuse sweating.
10. Arms and legs are bruised feeling, tired. They feel weary. Soreness is the key word. Prickling pain.
11. They take cold easily, especially in warm, moist air.
12. Eye injuries. Sore pain in eye. Eye feels weak, but is less inflamed; painful weakness of the eye. Feeling as if both eyes would be forced out of the head. Feels BETTER by pressing on them with the fingers but it is WORSE a few minutes afterward. (The person wants to press their fingers to the injured eye—but do not let them— nevertheless, this is a symptom to use this remedy.) Eye sore and painful under slight pressure. Eye inflamed, vessels greatly injected (congested). Swelling of eyeball and lid with bloodshot appearance of eye. Intense SORENESS.
13. Symptoms are WORSE from motion or movement, during the day, at rest, being out in open air, being touched, or in a warm room.

NOTES _____

_____

_____

_____

HYOSCYAMUS
(Henbane)

1. This remedy has been used in behavior disorders, strokes, hyperactivity, manic depression, paranoia, schizophrenia, seizure disorders, sexual disorders, recreational drug addictions, and others.
2. Talkative, suspicious, jealous, curses, lewd talk and behavior, dirty jokes, and a 'dirty mouth.' Obscene. Can be an exhibitionist; exposing genitals. Wants to be naked. Will do it for shock value.
3. Restless.
4. Manic and if angry, it turns to rage, which increases their strength. They may dance around with wild laughter and talking.
5. Cold, malicious, acts on the spur of the moment, impulsive.
6. Inclined to laugh at everything.
7. Mutters.
8. Talks to imaginary people or to the dead.
9. Plays with fingers almost incessantly. Gestures can be rhythmic and/or bizarre in appearance. Picks at things with their fingers, their clothes, bedding, etc.
10. Desire to masturbate in public; will handle sexual organs in public. Hypersexuality.
11. Foams at the mouth. Speech impaired. Tongue protrudes, can barely get it inside the mouth.
12. Face pale, flushed, dark red. Muscles twitch. Grimaces or makes ridiculous gestures with face.
13. Paranoid about being poisoned.
14. Pupils are dilated. Eyes sparkle and shine. Eyes roll about in the head. Spasmodic closing of eyelids. Aversion to light. Squints.
15. Symptoms are WORSE from their emotions, jealousy, being frightened, from being touched, cold temperatures, after eating, when lying down, in the evening and night, and experiencing unhappiness from a broken love affair/marriage.
16. Symptoms are BETTER from sitting up, from motion, being warm, and stooping.

SEE: **Stramonium** or **Tarentula Hispanica.**

NOTES _____

_____

_____

_____

_____

HYPERICUM
(St. John's-wort)

1. One of homeopathy's premier nerve and spinal column remedies. Any kind of spinal injury or nerve-related injury can respond well to this remedy (the genitalia, eyes, fingers, toes, tailbone or coccyx area, and tongue). Whiplash, a condition experienced after an auto accident where the muscles are in spasm, responds to this remedy. It is excellent for use in puncture wounds applied locally as in the case of insect bites or wild animal or domestic animal bites. Relieves pain after a surgical operation, for nerve injuries involving crushed fingers, toes, hands, and feet. The first nerve remedy to think of when the spinal column is injured, or in broken bones where there is nerve damage. This can also help in the 'phantom limb pain' experienced after an amputation, among others.

2. Excruciating pain characterized by tearing, sharp, shooting pains that are always worse if they try to lift their arms.

3. Paralytic weakness of affected part, with numbness, shooting, tingling, burning, or 'crawling' sensation in the injured area. Feels as if someone is sticking them with needles.

4. Pains shoot FROM the injured area, outward and extending accordingly.

5. Person lies on back, jerking their head backwards.

6. Joints feel bruised.

7. Pressure felt in sacrum (lower back) area.

8. After a tailbone injury, pain radiates UP the spine and DOWN the legs and arms. Jerking and twitching of muscles also can occur in the area of the back injury.

9. Symptoms are WORSE when there is jarring of the spine from shock, exertion, being touched, during a change of weather, during a fog, cold, dampness, from motion, being in a closed room, exposure to the weather, and after urinating.

10. Symptoms are BETTER when lying on face and bending backward.

NOTES _____

_____

_____

_____

_____

IGNATIA AMARA
(St. Ignatius Bean)

1. This remedy is often used with anger, hysteria and grief, convulsions, croup, anxiety, esophagus disorders, fainting, being frightened, locomotor ataxia (muscle uncoordination), psychological blindness, paralysis, sleep disorders, sore throats, among others. It is especially effective shortly after a trauma of any kind.

2. Person is hyperalert, nervous, apprehensive, rigid, trembling, or has erratic behavior.

3. Hysteria—but not always screaming, out-of-control symptoms—it can be a 'quiet' hysteria, too, where the person may be introspective, brooding, withdrawn, and incommunicative—so do not be fooled by this demeanor.

4. Sighing or sobbing a lot after the trauma. Their sighing is often and deep.

5. Violently repelled by cigarette, pipe, or cigar smoke.

6. Feelings are hurt very easily and they can become highly offended. Very defensive. Touchy. Prickly.

7. May be very doubting and suspicious of those trying to help, even rude.

8. The hysteria may later manifest as paralysis, numbness, or they go 'blind' after an accident (and their eyes were not injured), or after some traumatic grief/loss, or a limb(s) becomes paralyzed when there was no injury to it.

9. Does not want to cry; tries not to cry, but eventually gives into real, hard sobbing. Emotionally disconnected. Numbed out.

10. May continuously yawn (air hunger).

11. Symptoms are WORSE from being in the open, fresh air, cigarette odors, walking, standing, in the morning after breakfast, from drinking coffee, experiencing negative emotions (grief/trauma/worry/fright/shock), after losing a person or animal to death, or external warmth.

12. Symptoms are BETTER from swallowing, eating, and sitting near a warm stove.

NOTES _____

_____

_____

_____

_____

LACHESIS MUTA
(Bushmaster snake venom)

1. This remedy has been used for aneurysm, appendicitis, asthma, chilblains, cyanosis, epilepsy, fainting, heart disorders, high blood pressure, injuries, laryngismus, locomotor ataxia (muscle uncoordination), mumps, paralysis, poisonous insect bites/stings, poisonous snake bites, plague, pneumonia, pulmonary edema, strokes, sore throat, fevers, varicose veins, and wounds, among others.
2. Purple discoloration to the skin, bruised looking skin, red/violet or purple spots on the skin. Skin may also turn yellow, red, copper-colored spots, bluish-red or black looking.
3. Face is hot and flushed (red) looking.
4. Nosebleed.
5. Problems swallowing, especially liquids or saliva.
6. Does not want throat to be touched at all. Will pull away if you try to touch or examine it.
7. Hates tight-fitting clothes around neck and waist.
8. Does not want to be touched or have pressure applied to their skin.
9. Great anxiety, even phobia, with anxiousness, emotional intensity, and they may talk constantly.
10. Mentally, may show suspicion, jealousy, envy, or paranoia. They can be very aggressive and verbally abusive.
11. For hemorrhaging, poisonous bites or stings of insects, or poisonous snake bites and high blood pressure.
12. Arms and legs feel icy cold.
13. Symptoms are WORSE from sleeping, being touched, being out in direct sunlight, heat/temperature too high, wearing too tight a clothing, or consuming hot drinks of any kind.
13. Symptoms are BETTER from cold drinks, fresh air, being in the shade and out of direct sunlight, moderate temperature (70–75 degrees F), bathing the injured area, sitting bent, and warm applications.

SEE: **Crotalus Horridus, Elaps Corallinus**.

NOTES _____

_____

_____

_____

_____

LATRODECTUS MACTANS
(Black Widow)

1. This remedy has been used for poisonous spider bite, angina pectoris, or a heart attack, among others.
2. Severe abdominal pain, nausea, with sinking sensation in stomach region.
3. Cramps in the mid to lower back.
4. Violent pain extending from the chest (heart region) down the LEFT arm to the fingers. Numbness in the fingers. Sinking sensation in the chest. Cramping pain from chest to abdomen. Hands feel icy cold and numb.
5. Constant, pulsating pain in the eyes.
6. Extreme thirst. Vomits after drinking.
7. Fear of suffocation and dying. Anxiety about the heart. Will scream out in pain.
8. Symptoms are WORSE from the slightest movement. From any kind of exertion.
9. Symptoms are BETTER from sitting very still. No movement.

SEE: **Lachesis**.

NOTES _____

_____

_____

_____

_____

LAUROCERASUS
(Cherry Laurel)

1. This remedy has been used for cyanosis, bronchitis, pneumonia, "blue baby" condition shortly after being born, among others. It is one to think of in frostnip and frostbite situations. Or, in true hypothermia where the person is unconscious and frozen.
2. Coldness is not better from warmth being applied to it.
3. Blueness (cyanosis) to the skin.
4. Skin is cool and black and blue looking. Toes and fingers become 'knotty' feeling. Cold, clammy feet and legs. Veins in hands are distended.
5. No reaction from the person if shaken or spoken to, face pale, blue, and the surface of it is cold.
6. Internal feeling of coldness. Tongue is cold. There may be sensations of heat in certain parts of the body, here and there.
7. Tendency to ooze blood that is bright red and mixed with gelatinous clots.
8. Gasping for breath, puts hand over heart.
9. Symptoms are WORSE sitting up, with exertion, from cold temperatures or cold foods/fluids, on stooping, and in the evening and at night.
10. Symptoms are BETTER from lying with head low and laying down. Sometimes, the opposite, where person is worse sitting up.

SEE: **Agaricus Muscarius** and **Petroleum** in frostnip/frostbite and hypothermia situations.

NOTES _____

_____

_____

_____

_____

LEDUM
(Marsh Tea)

1. This remedy has been used for bruising, bleeding (blood is dark, venous color), bites, stings, and wounds (puncture type in particular) that are always BETTER with ice packs, cold cloth, or cold bathing of the affected part.
2. Person is cold and chilly, but cold bathing or application makes them feel better.
3. Face may be mottled, bloated, or puffy looking.
4. Bruises are swollen and purple colored.
5. May be very cross, irritable, or surly.
6. The wound site itself feels COLD to the person.
7. Symptoms are BETTER with cold applications, ice applied to region, and being out in cold air, placing feet in cold water, or lying down.
8. Symptoms are WORSE at night, from the heat of a bed, warm covers, warm stove, or warm air. Worse with motion.

SEE: **Lachesis**.

NOTES _____

_____

_____

_____

_____

MOSCHUS

(Deer musk)

1. This remedy has been used for asthma, fainting (psychogenic shock), hysterical behavior, hysterical convulsions, and heart palpitations, among others.
2. Fits of anger along with scolding until the person is literally "blue in the face."
3. Fainting caused by hysteria or some emotional, overwhelming situation or crisis.
4. Anxiety; fear of impending death.
5. Asthma caused by hysteria; spasms of the chest are frightening and come on suddenly and severely. Wants to take a deep breath. Difficult breathing. Chest feels oppressed. Feels as if lungs are paralyzed. Spasms of the epiglottis (throat region).
6. Lips turn blue.
7. Uncontrollable laughter.
8. Mentally hurried, awkward, drops things from hands.
9. Raves, scolds, talks excitedly, may exhibit violent anger.
10. Cough ceases, mucus cannot be expectorated.
11. A sensation of a ball in the throat, which causes hysteria.
12. Symptoms are WORSE from becoming excited, being cold, in open air, from pressure, motion, after a meal, or during a meal.
13. Symptoms are BETTER from being out in open air, rubbing, lying down, and being still.

NOTES _____

_____

_____

_____

_____

NUX MOSCHATA
(Nutmeg)

1. This remedy has been used in Alzheimer's disease, colic, narcolepsy, organic brain syndrome, petit mal epilepsy, and fainting (psychogenic shock), among others.
2. Fainting with heart palpitations from the sight of blood or from a food allergy.
3. Appears bewildered, as if in a dream, mood is changeable, memory is impaired. Spacy. Absent-minded.
4. Forgetful. Forgets why they have come into a room. Thoughts seem to vanish or wander.
5. Fear of the sight of blood (which induces fainting).
6. May appear sleepy or very drowsy or say they have an overpowering urge to go to sleep.
7. Fainting due to heart failure.
8. Hands and feet are cold.
9. All mucous membranes are very dry (mouth, throat, nose, etc.) and so is their skin. They have 'cotton' in their mouth. Tongue is dry and may adhere to the top of their mouth. Tongue may be numb feeling and thick. No desire for water despite this situation.
10. Will smack their lips.
11. Heart feels as if it is trembling or fluttering. As if a hand gripped their heart. Palpitations.
12. Symptoms are WORSE from cold bathing, dampness, windy conditions, drafts, fog, eating cold food, allowing their feet to get cold, change of season, during the summer, and in hot weather. They are worse from their emotions, from excitement, exertion, from being jarred, from mental exertion or shock, from overheating, drinking milk, or shaking their head.
13. Symptoms are BETTER from moist, warm heat being applied, being in a warm room, and being in dry weather.

NOTES _____

_____

_____

_____

_____

NUX VOMICA

(Poison Nut)

1. This remedy helps with food poisoning, gall bladder attacks, asthma, digestive disorders, cerebral vascular accidents (stroke), and from recreational drug overdoses, among others.
2. Weight and pain in the stomach.
3. Stomach region very sensitive to pressure.
4. Stomach area bloated or swollen feeling. May feel as if a stone is in the stomach.
5. Nausea and vomiting with a lot of gagging or retching.
6. Violent vomiting.
7. Food lies like a heavy knot in the stomach.
8. Wants to vomit, but cannot.
9. Stomach pains that are worse with tight clothes around their waist.
10. Cramping, sharp pains felt in the abdomen.
11. Symptoms are WORSE with tight clothing, cold temperature, from drinking coffee or alcoholic beverages, narcotics, recreational drugs, mental exertion, disturbed sleep, odors, noise, being touched, hearing music, and overeating.
12. Symptoms are BETTER from taking a nap, resting during damp, wet weather, strong pressure, wrapping head, hot drinks, drinking milk, and lying on side.

SEE: **Tarentula Hispanica**, if a drug overdose.

NOTES _____

_____

_____

_____

_____

OPIUM

NOTE: This is a potentized homeopathic remedy that has no crude opium substance in the 30C pellets or dilution. It must be dispensed via prescription by a licensed physician in the United States. Consult your homeopath.

1. This remedy has been utilized in coma, unconsciousness, strokes, convulsions, narcolepsy, head injury, eclampsia (high blood pressure in pregnant women with convulsions), and strokes, among others.
2. Speech thick and nearly incoherent.
3. Fear and shock. Shock brought on by some horrific fright or trauma.
4. Shock symptoms of drowsiness, stupor, or alternating states of consciousness and/or awareness.
5. Face flushed a deep red or mottled purple.
6. Pupils constricted or dilated.
7. Convulsions.
8. Labored, snoring breath; pulse slow and full.
9. Drooping jaw.
10. Tongue paralysis.
11. Eyes heavy and half closed.
12. Stupor alternating with restlessness.
13. Delusional.
14. Urine retention.
15. Cheyne-Stokes Respiration in coma.
16. Symptoms WORSE from anxiety, fear, from their own or other people's emotional outbursts (joy, shame, fright, etc.), odor, alcohol, during and after sleep, and from any type of stimulant (alcohol, coffee, addictive/recreational drugs).
17. Symptoms BETTER from cold, uncovering, and constant walking.

NOTES _____

_____

_____

_____

_____

PETROLEUM
(Crude rock-oil)

1. This remedy has been used for asthma, motion sickness, and otitis media and should be considered in cases of frostnip and frostbite, among others.
2. Skin is dry and cracked, and cracks will be deep and bloody.
3. Skin is unhealthy looking (there is a 'dirty' look to it) and it suppurates (leaks lymph fluid) from cracked regions.
4. Cold sensation to the skin after scratching the area.
5. Itching is very intense and strong.
6. Itching is always worse at night, especially in the warmth of a bed.
7. Cracking at the fingertips and possibly cracks in the palm of the hands.
8. Affected area may be moist, itchy, and burning. Brown spots are present.
9. Skin may be dirty, hard, rough, and thickened like leather.
10. Skin gets raw, festers, and will NOT heal—and is worse in the folds of the limbs (inside of elbow, behind the knees).
11. Thick, greenish crusts, burning, itching, redness, raw, and cracks and bleeds easily.
12. Skin may itch, burn, and become purple colored.
13. Symptoms are WORSE from being exposed to dampness or damp conditions, in the winter, cold weather, changing weather, and passive motion (riding in a car).
14. Symptoms are BETTER from warm air (blowing breath on frozen area), lying with head high, and in dry weather.

SEE: **Agaricus Muscarius** and **Laurocerasus** for frostnip, frostbite, and hypothermia.

NOTES _____

_____

_____

_____

_____

PHOSPHORUS

1. This remedy has been used for angina, anxiety, asthma, congestive heart failure, eye-related injuries, Hyphema, croup, nosebleed, petit mal epilepsy, phobia disorders, pneumonia, respiratory infection, valvular heart disorders, among others.
2. One of the premier hemorrhaging remedies.
3. For nosebleeds.
4. Easily reassured by person in charge.
5. Easily frightened by suggestions—be careful what you say around them; they become overwrought and anxious.
6. Needs company or people or attention at all times, especially during an injury or trauma. Shock can be ameliorated to a degree by touching them with a reassuring hand.
7. Easily dehydrated.
8. For use in collapsed and debilitating states such as shock and hemorrhaging.
9. For strokes and cerebral accidents with paralysis on one side of the body.
10. Detached retina, glaucoma, and other eye trauma (bleeding). Sensation as if everything is covered with a mist or veil or something is pulled tightly over the eyes. Eyes feel "stiff." Pupil(s) are contracted (black pinpoint in field of eye). Greenish or reddish halo about candle light (light bulb). Letters appear red.
11. Thrombosis (blood clot) of retinal vessels and degenerative changes in the retina. Retinal trouble with lights and hallucination of vision.
12. Pain in eyes, pressure in eyes as from a grain of sand. Eyes itch. Pressure in the eye as if it is going to be pushed or pressed out of the socket. Shooting, smarting, heat and burning sensation in the eye. Pressing, burning pain in the eyes. Tearing, especially in open air and facing the wind.
13. Congestion of blood in the eye. Redness of sclera and conjunctiva. Yellowish colored sclera. Everything seems to have a gray veil. As if a black veil is before the eyes. May see many colors when there is only one color. Black reflections or sparks and black spots before the eye.
14. Bleeding peptic ulcers. Will have bright red blood or 'coffee-ground' colored blood.
15. Desire for cold drinks.
16. Angina pectoris where pains come on due to stress and they are worse lying on their left side and better from cold drinks and fluids.
17. Postoperative vomiting from anesthesia.
18. Water is thrown up as soon as it warms up in stomach.

19. Symptoms are WORSE from being touched, physical/mental exertion, warm food or drink, getting wet in hot weather, in the evening, lying on their left or painful side, climbing stairs, from a change of weather, from talking, odors, warm food, suffering from loss of fluids (perspiration, bleeding, vomiting, diarrhea, urination, etc.), and during a thunderstorm.

20. Symptoms are BETTER by being in the dark, lying on their right side, eating cold food, being in cooling/cold air (also air conditioning), being out in open air or near an opened window, washing with cold water, sleeping, being massaged, or sitting.

NOTES _____

_____

_____

_____

_____

PYROGENIUM

(Scraping from rotted meat)

1. This remedy has been used for septic shock conditions and symptoms, abscesses, flu, blood poisoning, ptomaine poisoning (food poisoning), high fever with delirium, wounds, or sepsis in general of any kind, among others.
2. Pulse is bounding and hard—out of proportion with the temperature—or the reverse.
3. Ground or bed or floor feels too hard.
4. Frequent urination.
5. Throbbing pulsation in blood veins and arteries. Forehead bathed in a cold sweat.
6. Mind is full of anxiety or crazy notions.
7. Restless, talks or whispers to self, even while asleep.
8. Cannot tell whether they are dreaming or awake.
9. Red circles on cheeks.
10. Face can be burning, yellowish, very red, pale, sunken, bathed in cold sweat or greenish looking. Perspiration is COLD feeling.
11. Great thirst for small quantities of cold drinks that if consumed will be vomited right back up.
12. Heart palpitations made worse by moving around.
13. Heart beat so loud the person can hear it. A throbbing is felt in the head and ears, preventing sleep.
14. Heart feels too large or too full of blood. Feels as if the heart is pumping out cold water.
15. Sweating does NOT lower the temperature. Sweats without relief.
16. High fever with sore limbs and delirium. Temperature rises rapidly.
17. So cold that they cannot get warm or close enough to a stove or fire.
18. Shivers and moves around restlessly.
19. Staggers around upon rising. Dizziness if they sit up in bed or chair.
20. When a wound refuses to heal, think of Pyrogenium.
21. Symptoms are WORSE in cold, dampness, when in motion, sitting up, or moving their eyes.
22. Symptoms are BETTER from heat, hot bath, hot drinks, pressure, stretching, changing position, hard rocking, or walking.

NOTES _____

_____

_____

_____

RHUS TOXICODENDRON
(Poison Oak/Ivy)

1. This remedy has been used for arthritis, asthma, behavior disorder, bronchitis, whiplash (cervical injury), bed wetting, rheumatism, shingles, sprains, tendonitis, poisoning by oak and ivy, among others.
2. Skin is itchy and is better from hot water application.
3. Thickened skin from long-standing skin disorders.
4. Dark, reddish splotches on skin.
5. Skin is hot and swollen, and the itching is intense. It is a dry, hot burning that is worse on hairy parts of the body.
6. Suppuration from skin eruptions that scale. Sensitive to cold air.
7. Symptoms are WORSE from cold, rainy weather, after a rain, at night, exposure to wet, cold air, to a draft, getting chilled or being hot and sweaty, at the beginning of motion, at rest, before a storm, and from prolonged sitting after exertion.
8. Symptoms are BETTER from continued motion, heat, a hot shower or bath, warm application to the injured area, stretching limbs, changing position, and walking.

NOTES _____

_____

_____

_____

_____

RUTA GRAVEOLENS
(Garden Rue)

1. This remedy has been extremely useful in connective tissue ailments, rheumatism, anxiety disorders, straining tendons, tendonitis, neuralgia, low back pain, fibromyalgia conditions, the wrist joints (such as carpal tunnel syndrome), eyestrain, sciatica, and 'bruised' bones and broken bones (especially rib fractures). NOTE: Major symptoms are BETTER with rest. Even the smallest of movement aggravates the symptoms 10 times more.
2. Cracking sound in joints.
3. Pain and stiffness in hands and fingers.
4. Legs give out when rising from a chair.
5. Paralytic weakness of legs after spraining the back.
6. Stiffness felt around injury or throughout the body.
7. Anxiety about death with a high fever or if overheated.
8. Tendons feel sore.
9. Knees give out.
10. Ankle swollen from strain or injury.
11. Bursitis.
12. Easily tired from physical exertion of any kind.
13. Soreness felt on part of body that is laid upon.
14. Restless.
15. Eyestrain from using the eyes too much (reading, needlepoint, computers, etc.). Burning and redness of eyes.
16. Overuse of tendons that causes fibrosis.
17. Nodular (nodes) growths due to overuse.
18. Symptoms are WORSE from movement of any kind, climbing up or down hills/stairs, cold, wet weather, or dampness.
19. Symptoms are BETTER from lying on back, warmth, rubbing or scratching the area.

NOTES _____

_____

_____

_____

SAMBUCUS NIGRA

(Elder)

1. This remedy has been used for allergies, asthma, bronchitis, croup, laryngospasm, and pertussis, among others.
2. Constant, nonstop coughing that comes on about midnight, with crying (if baby or young child) and shortness of breath.
3. Child awakes suddenly, nearly suffocating, sits up, turns blue. Cannot exhale or breathe out. May have a loose, choking cough.
4. Hoarseness with tenacious mucus in the larynx that refuses to be coughed up and out.
5. Spasmodic croup. Turning blue during seizure.
6. Hands turn blue, feet are icy cold, and child has debilitating night sweats while in coughing mode. After coughing is done, perspiration disappears. Perspiration over entire body—except the head.
7. Heaviness, constriction in chest with heart palpitations. May be awakened from sleep with terrible, constricting feeling around heart and chest.
8. Cold hands and feet—but rest of body is warm.
9. Infant who breastfeeds will let go of the nipple; nose is blocked up and cannot breathe.
10. Wants to remain covered up—actually dreads being uncovered.
11. Symptoms are WORSE from consuming cold drinks, eating fruit, during sleep, lying down on bed, on left side, from motion, about midnight or 2 am to 3 am, being uncovered, from dry, cold air, and if head is low, they must sit up to regain breath.
12. Symptoms are BETTER from sitting up in bed.

SEE: **Spongia Tosta**.

NOTES _____

_____

_____

_____

_____

SPONGIA TOSTA

(Roasted Sponge)

1. This remedy is used for asthma, croup, bronchitis, asthma, laryngismus, and angina, among others.
2. Croup is worse BEFORE midnight.
3. Cough is created by a tickling or irritation in throat or chest.
4. Cough is dry—like a saw going through wood, a seal's bark, or a barking, harsh sound.
5. Anxiety that they are going to die from suffocation.
6. Dryness of the mucous membranes of the tongue, throat, larynx, and windpipe.
7. Anxiety with difficulty in breathing.
8. Mucus cannot be raised or coughed out of body; stubborn and must be swallowed.
9. Weakness felt in chest; they can barely talk. Oppression and heat felt in chest. Burning, rawness, and soreness felt in chest.
10. Constriction felt in throat, with tickling and dryness.
11. Pain felt in throat when coughing, talking, touching the area, or trying to speak.
12. Hoarseness. Voice gives way when speaking.
13. Throat feels as if it is burning and stinging. Dryness. Swallows small sips of water with great difficulty.
14. Symptoms are WORSE climbing up stairs, before midnight, from experiencing a cold, dry wind or draft, from raising arms, from exertion of any kind, from touching the affected area, when walking, stooping, rising, or talking.
15. Symptoms are BETTER when walking downstairs, resting in a horizontal position, eating or drinking warm food or fluids, keeping head low when lying down. Frosty weather helps cough.

SEE: **Sambucus Nigra.**

NOTES _____

_____

_____

_____

_____

STANNUM
(Tin)

1. This remedy is useful in nervous system or respiratory disorders and in ailments where weakness or depletion are obvious. The symptoms come on very slowly, but surely. Also, where symptoms 'hang fire' and the person is never able to get rid of the cough or upper respiratory infection. It was used for tuberculosis in the 19th century. Chronic obstructive pulmonary diseases may respond well to this remedy, but a professional homeopath needs to decide this for the patient. Excellent for chest injuries (after they've seen a physician), asthma, bronchitis, chronic fatigue syndrome, pneumonia, or a reoccurring fever/cough, among others.
2. Breathing is difficult or weak. Shortness of breath with slightest of exertion (talking).
3. Hollow and empty feeling in the chest.
4. Cannot speak.
5. Mucus is plentiful, with a sweet/salty taste to it, and is usually a pale yellow color. Can be offensive smelling, too.
6. Coughing is hard, painful, and deep with green, thick mucus spit up or coughed up. Must hold chest when they cough (because it is so deep and the pain is present). May cough, gag, and then vomit.
7. Cough is excited by talking, singing, laughing.
8. Legs give out when attempting to sit down.
9. Knees are tremulous and weak.
10. Symptoms are WORSE when using voice, from cold temperature/weather, around 10 am, with gentle motion, lying on their right side, from consuming warm drink, walking downstairs or upstairs, and being touched.
11. Symptoms are BETTER when walking, but must rest soon thereafter, from pressure (hand on chest) and being in open air, lying across something hard, from coughing or expectorating the mucus, from rapid motion or bending double.

NOTES _____

_____

_____

_____

_____

STAPHYSAGRIA
(Stavesacre)

1. This remedy has been used for cerebral vascular accidents (stroke), post-surgical pain, strabismus, and severe pain following an abdominal operation, among others.
2. Diarrhea with straining after drinking cold water.
3. Constipation with enlarged prostate.
4. Abdominal pain felt after experiencing anger.
5. Peptic ulcer.
6. Trembling from anger or emotions.
7. Paralysis after cerebral accident (stroke/aneurysm).
8. Sleepy during the day, but sleepless at night.
9. Bed wetting.
10. Prostate enlargement with retained urine.
11. Backache; worse in morning after rising.
12. Symptoms are WORSE from getting angry (the person usually does not express or show their anger, but swallows it, instead), being humiliated, shamed, from grief, from touching the injured area, from loss of fluids (sweating, vomiting, diarrhea, urination, bleeding, etc.), consuming cold drinks, and stretching the affected part.
13. Symptoms are BETTER after breakfast, warmth, and rest at night.

NOTES _____

_____

_____

_____

_____

STRAMONIUM
(Thorn Apple)

1. This remedy is often used in ADD, behavioral disorders, strokes, febrile convulsions, head injury, hyperactive children, manic depression, phobic disorders, schizophrenia, seizure disorders, stammering, recreational drug addiction, among others.
2. Rage and violence—this person can commit murder.
3. May strike out, bite, hit, kick, strangle someone—any kind of violent, murderous behavior.
4. Great fear of the darkness; they must have light and company.
5. Does not want to be left alone—needs company.
6. Impassioned speech, earnest, beseeching, and ceaseless talking. A nonstop talker. Can be foul-mouthed, swears, and can be lewd.
7. Delirium with talking, laughing, singing, swearing, praying, and rhyming.
8. Sees ghosts, hears voices, and talks with spirits.
9. Eyes are wide, staring, and open; pupils are dilated.
10. Dribbling of saliva from corners of mouth.
11. May stammer. Cannot swallow on account of a spasm. A chewing motion to the mouth.
12. Filled with terror—fixed ideas—compulsive/obsessive behavior.
13. If they see water or hear it running, they become 10 times more fearful and anxious.
14. Hallucinations of all kinds that terrify them; wildly excitable. They hallucinate that they are taller than everyone else, that there are two of themselves (double), or there is a part missing from themselves.
15. Rapid changes from euphoria and joy to sadness. Manic depression or manic behavior.
16. Symptoms are WORSE when they see shining objects (mirror, the glint off a piece of metal, sunlight reflecting off a window, etc.), on cloudy days, from being touched, left alone, in the dark, when alone after sleep or when swallowing, hearing water running or seeing water, and being out in the sun.
17. Symptoms are BETTER from being in a brightly lit room, having company, and being warm.

SEE: **Hyoscyamus** or **Tarentula Hispanica**.

NOTES _____

_____

_____

_____

SYMPHYTUM
(Comfrey)

1. This remedy has been used for broken bones, torn ligaments/tendons, or any joint injury that will not heal up with the use of other homeopathic remedies. Also used for bone cancer, stone bruises, or anything pertaining to the periosteum (the tissue around the bone that nourishes it), bone injuries that do not heal, eye injuries, bone pains that continue long after healing, or phantom limb pain experienced after an amputation. Also of use if a breast receives blunt trauma. It has also been used in sprains, strains, osteoporosis, or decay of the spinal vertebrae, among others. Excellent for any injury to the eyeball.
2. Pricking, jagged, or sticking pain around the injury.
3. Inflammation, hardness, redness, and swelling of a bone after it has been injured.
4. Bone feels sore.
5. Symptoms are always WORSE after the injury, from being touched, and from walking. Sitting causes pain around the belly button; stooping causes weight in forehead.

NOTES _____

_____

_____

_____

_____

TARENTULA HISPANICA
(Spanish Spider)

1. This remedy has been used in behavior disorders, hyperactivity, mania, restless leg syndrome, and angina, among others. Should be thought of in poisoning from plants that cause central nervous system disturbance, among others.
2. Person is very hurried, restless, intense, and excitable.
3. Loves music and will dance around.
4. Does not want to be touched.
5. Very cunning and manipulative; will lie, is destructive (will break things, tear them down, or throw items at you), will rage at you during a manic episode, and has the power of 10 men; has tremendous passion, extremism, violence, and can kill. Can be hyperactive, stubborn, and disobedient, with laughing and wild, inexplicable behavior. Can be very destructive.
6. Face is fiery red, bloated, an expression of terror; may be wrinkled.
7. Feels as if a thousand needles are pricking them in the head. May rub head constantly or pull or tug at hair because it makes their headache feel better.
8. Hands and feet are cold and moist. Arms and hands in constant, nonstop motion. Legs are in constant, restless motion. Person cannot sit quietly at all. Something is always moving on them; whether tapping a finger, a foot, or moving restlessly about.
9. Legs are numb feeling. Twitching, jerking, and weakness in legs; cannot walk and will not obey. Soles of feet itch.
10. Skin may be dark red or purplish looking. Bruised spots on skin. Swelling of the skin and tissue.
11. Symptoms are WORSE from being touched, when it is cold and damp, in the evening, at night, hearing noises, washing head, or placing hands under cold water.
12. Symptoms are BETTER from being out in open air, from listening to music, from pressure or rubbing the affected part, relaxing, sweating, moving around, and taking a warm shower or bath.

SEE: **Stramonium** or **Hyoscyamus**.

NOTES _____

_____

_____

_____

_____

URTICA URENS
(Stinging Nettle)

1. This remedy has been used for fever, gout, rheumatism, first and second degree burns, insect bites and stings, and serious sunburn, among others.
2. Injured skin has a stinging, burning pain along with an exquisite sensitivity to it. May have a scalding sensation to it.
3. Especially indicated for genital burns.
4. Serious sunburn that has intense burning and itching.
5. Itching, raised, and red blotched or nettle-rash looking skin. Burning heat with injury and violent itching. Can also have prickly heat/itching.
6. Symptoms are WORSE from winter air, humid/cool air (air conditioning, also), or cool bathing, by being touched, violent exertion, after sleeping, application of water to injury, or being exposed to a cool, moist atmosphere.
7. Symptoms are BETTER from lying down.

NOTES _____

_____

_____

_____

_____

VERATRUM ALBUM
(White Hellebore)

1. This remedy has been used for behavioral disorders, hyperactivity, mania, manic depression, neuralgia, seizures, and may be of use in neurogenic shock cases where spinal cord injury is apparent, among others.
2. Dizziness with vomiting and a cold sweat. Projectile vomiting. It is worse by drinking fluids or with the least movement.
3. Headache with icy coldness, especially on the top of the head. Cold sweat on forehead only.
4. Internal coldness—they feel as if ice water is flowing in their veins.
5. Weakness and any collapsed state, especially during vomiting or diarrhea.
6. Mentally, they may doing meaningless, repetitive tasks; hyperactive, rude, critical, psychotic behavior, religious, excessive praying, sullen or indifferent, hangs head down and broods.
7. Icy coldness on the tip of the nose.
8. Thirst for cold water that is vomited up as soon as it is swallowed.
9. Face is extremely pale, blue, and they are cold and collapsing. Face may look deathly pale, pinched or distorted or frowning or a terrified look on it. Lips blue and they hang down.
10. Skin blue, cold, clammy, and with a cold sweat. Skin is flabby, without elasticity.
11. Symptoms are WORSE from exertion, cold drinks, wet, cold weather, at night, from being touched or pressure applied to injured area.
12. Symptoms are BETTER (if a child) from being carried, warmth, a covering over them, hot drinks, and lying down.

NOTES _____

_____

_____

_____

_____

APPENDICES

A. Ordering the Advanced Homeopathic First Aid Kit

B. Emergency Supplies for Every Household

C. Homeopathic Information and Contacts

D. History of Homeopathy

E. Making Dilutions from Homeopathic Pellets

F. Other Books by the Author

G. Blue Turtle Flower and Gem Essences

H. Seminar and Workshop Information

I. Cara Help! Software Information

J. Flower and Gem Essence Consultant Training Information

Appendix A

ORDERING THE "ADVANCED HOMEOPATHIC FIRST AID KIT"
(Advertisement)

The Advanced First Aid Kit can be purchased from the following vendor:

Hahnemann Pharmacy   Phone: 510-527-3003
1940 4th Street   Toll Free: 888-427-6422
San Rafael, CA 94901

Kit includes 50 homeopathic remedies in 2 dram sizes at 30C potency. The price is $119.95 plus shipping and tax in California. Call Monday through Friday, 9 am to 5 pm, PST.

Appendix B

EMERGENCY SUPPLIES FOR EVERY HOUSEHOLD

The supplies that you should have available at home:

1. Protective latex or vinyl gloves.
2. CPR Microshield (mouth barrier with one-way valve).
3. Rubbing alcohol.
4. Safety pins.
5. Elastic bandages.
6. Knife.
7. Scissors that can cut through clothes to expose a wound site.
8. Thermometer.
9. Sterile dressings/bandages, compresses 4 x 4.
10. Butterfly bandages.
11. Adhesive tape.
12. Tweezers.
13. Plastic wrap, plastic bags, and foil.
14. Activated charcoal in case of poisoning.
15. Syrup of Ipecac.
16. Sterile water.
17. Saline solution.
18. Fels Naptha soap.
19. Meat tenderizer.

The emergency homeopathic supplies you should have at home:

1. Calendula tincture.
2. Hypericum tincture.
3. Arnica oil (never put in an open wound and never drink it—to be used externally only on UNBROKEN skin).
4. Advanced Homeopathic First Aid Kit (see Appendix A).

Appendix C

HOMEOPATHIC INFORMATION AND CONTACTS

National Center for Homeopathy
801 North Fairfax Street, Suite 306
Alexandria, VA 22314-1757
Phone: (703) 548-7790
Fx: (703) 548-7792
Email: nchinfo@igc.apc.org
Internet: http://www.healthy.net (this home page provides valuable information on what homeopathy is and a directory of available homeopaths by state) or try http://www.dimensional/~stevew.

NCH will provide brochures, for a minimal fee, on what homeopathy is, as well as a directory of homeopaths in the United States/Canada. They will provide information on the nearest NCH-affiliated homeopathic study group so that you can learn more about homeopathy. NCH also provides yearly courses for professionals and consumers in homeopathy. Call or write for details.

JOIN NCH!

If you want to join this organization, the membership fee is $40 or $55 USD if outside the USA and Canada. Please send a check to the above address. You will receive the directory of homeopaths in the United States and Canada, as well as information on the nearest homeopathic pharmacy, affiliated study groups, and more. You will also receive a monthly newsletter from NCH chock full of information on this wonderful alternative medicine.

STATES THAT HAVE LICENSED OR CERTIFIED HOMEOPATHY:

Arizona, Connecticut and Nevada have state licensing boards for homeopaths.

Oregon: Homeopathic Academy of Naturopathic Physicians, 12132 SE Foster Place, Portland, OR 97266. They have a national listing of their DHANP graduates. (503) 761-3298.

American Board of Homeotherapeutics, 801 North Fairfax St., Suite 306, Alexandria, VA 22314. Open to MDs and DOs; they are awarded a DHt. 1-703-548-7790.

Appendix D

HISTORY OF HOMEOPATHY

For those who are interested in knowing a bit more about the history of homeopathy in the United States, Julian Winston has made a one-hour video called *The Faces of Homeopathy*. This narrative, enhanced by a music track and more than 300 images of people and places, traces the history from the inception of homeopathy in Germany in the late 1700s through the rise of homeopathic study groups in the mid 1980s. The video is available from the National Center for Homeopathy or from selected homeopathic booksellers.

Several people have asked Julian to expand upon his video—to give more details to the presentation. These requests will be answered in late 1998 or early 1999 with the publication of *The Faces of Homeopathy*, a 300-page illustrated coffee table book that documents the rise, the decline, and the resurgence of homeopathy in the United States.

The latest illustrated history was written by W.H. King in 1905. The new book will include a short history of homeopathy in each state, and an exposition of homeopathy in the United States from the late 1930s until the 1990s—a time that has never been adequately written about.

Julian also maintains a database of more than 20,000 graduates of homeopathic schools and homeopathic practitioners in the United States from 1850 until the mid 1960s.

For information concerning historical matters in homeopathy, Julian may be contacted by e-mail at jwinston@actrix.gen.nz or by post at PO Box 510156, Tawa 6006, New Zealand.

Appendix E

MAKING DILUTIONS FROM HOMEOPATHIC PELLETS

1. Choose a bottle. I would suggest going to your local pharmacy and buying some one-ounce eyedropper bottles.

2. Both eyedroppers and bottles must be sterilized. Unscrew the eyedropper cap from the bottle and place them in boiling water. Cover and boil for 20 minutes. Set them out to air dry.

3. When the bottle has cooled, do the following: Pour out 10–15 pellets from the bottle of the remedy you want to make into a fluid dilution into a teaspoon. Do not touch them with your fingers. Transfer them carefully to the awaiting sterilized eyedropper bottle.

4. Depending upon how LONG you want the dilution to last, you may put in more or less brandy as a base for it. Alcohol "stores" things. The more brandy, the longer the shelf life. If you can't use alcohol, then vinegar is best, but its shelf life is very limited and it must be kept in the refrigerator at all times. You can take a brandy-based solution with you anywhere and it doesn't have to be refrigerated. Generally speaking, I would use half brandy and half water (city/well or distilled is fine).

5. Cap it and be sure to write on the bottle what the remedy is and the potency of the remedy: Aconitum Napellus 30C, for example. If you have a brandy-based dilution, store it in a cool, dark place (like a pantry). Never put it out in direct sunlight. Storage in a room of a house is fine. If it is made with a vinegar base, keep it in a refrigerator. Usually, green mold will grow in it eventually and when it does, it must be replaced.

6. You may want to make up all of your pellet remedies into dilutions, and that would take 48 bottles. Never make more than one at a time. Do not have two different homeopathic remedy bottles open at the same time. Store them together. If you have a carrier of some kind, take them with you on vacation, picnics, travels, etc.

7. The pellets in the bottle will dissolve within 2 hours. Before you use the remedy, shake it up a little, then open it up and use the eyedropper to place the liquid appropriately as outlined in this book.

8. To apply a drop behind the ear or on the underside of the wrist, place a pair of latex or rubber gloves on before you GENTLY rub it on the skin. If you do not wear gloves for protection you will also absorb the remedy and under perfect conditions, you do not want to do this. If you have no gloves, just place a drop on the skin and rub it in GENTLY with the tip of the eyedropper itself.

Poisons That Heal. $14.95. Eileen Nauman. For anyone, including the homeopathic practitioner, this book is about well-known and exotic epidemics that do and may, in the future, affect us globally. How prepared are you? Eileen has shared homeopathic remedies for flu, colds, measles, mumps, Hanta virus, whooping cough, Lyme disease, strep-A flesh-eating bacteria, Ebola, and more. She also discusses remedies to support menopause, depression, and other emotional ailments. There is additional information on homeopathic remedies for first aid situations, understanding homeopathy, building your own homeopathic kit, information on headaches and acne, and information and help through particular flower and gem essences.

Path of the Mystic. $11.95. Ai Gvhdi Waya (Eileen Nauman). "Our best teachers are inside ourselves." That is the message that Eileen wants to impart through a series of true Native American stories that she has experienced and written about. Through her journey of discovery you may discover ways to access your own teachers from within. She advocates self-empowerment, so that you listen to yourself, instead of running to somebody else who may or may not have your best interests at heart. Walk the path of the mystic and understand how you can do it on a daily basis too.

Appendix F

Other Books by
Eileen Nauman, DHM, DIHom (UK), EMT

Now available from Blue Turtle Publishing
P.O. Box 2513, Cottonwood, AZ 86326
E-mail: docbones@sedona.net.

Soul Recovery and Extraction. $9.95. Ai Gvhdi Waya (Eil
Nauman). An ancient Native American healing technique, shamani
and how it can be used today to help us heal not only wounds of
spirit, but also emotional, mental, and physical wounds. Part East
Cherokee, Eileen's father was a shaman and trained her and her broth
Gary Gent, to carry on this family healing tradition. Case histori
explanation of the technique, and a directory of shamanic facilitators a
included.

Medical Astrology. $29.95. One of the world's best references on th
topic, Part I discusses the astrology of medicine. Part 2 offers a wealth o
health information, including vitamins, minerals, Bach flower remedies
homeopathic remedies, natural (flower/gem) essences, and much more.
This book can be read and understood by both astrologers and non
astrologers.

Bach Flower Remedies and Astrology. $6.95. A guide to using Dr.
Bach's flower remedies, for the astrologer as well as the non-astrologer.
Assignment of zodiac signs, planets, and houses to the 38 remedies. An
indispensable book that should be in everyone's medicine cabinet. Easy
to understand and use.

Colored Stones and Healing. $4.95. Eileen Nauman and Ruth Gent.
The authors draw upon their Eastern Cherokee upbringing and
experience, and share Apache medicine woman Oh Shinnah Fast Wolf's
technique for healing with precious and semiprecious gemstones. More
than 50 stones are given, with their healing properties, their symbols,
and which chakras they are associated with.

Beauty in Bloom: Homeopathy to Support Menopause. $29.95. August
1999. This self-help book about menopause as a natural occurrence in
every woman's life gives alternatives to hormone replacement therapy
and explains why you should consider homeopathy as a viable option.
Specific homeopathic remedies for every symptom of menopause are
detailed. Choose the remedy you need. The last third of your life can be
the best years of your life—naturally, and without deadly, cancer-
causing HRT drugs. There are choices, and Eileen gives them to you.

Appendix G

BLUE TURTLE NATURAL ESSENCES

Flower and gem essences made by Eileen Nauman. She uses these in her homeopathic practice. Much gentler than homeopathic remedies and excellent for sensitive individuals.

FREE CATALOG: Write to Blue Turtle Publishing, PO Box 2513, Cotton-wood, AZ 86326. Or, E-mail to docbones@sedona.net and request a copy (add your postal address).

Want to be a prover on a flower or gem essence proving? Contact Eileen for details at the above street or E-mail address.

Appendix H

EILEEN NAUMAN SEMINAR AND
WORKSHOP INFORMATION

Each year, Eileen gives five-day seminars on the following topics in Sedona, Arizona. If you are interested in any of these training seminars, please write her at Eileen Nauman, PO Box 2513, Cottonwood, AZ 86326 for a free brochure or E-mail her at docbones@sedona.net and provide your postal address.

1. **Flower and Gem Essence seminar.** How to make, create, and use flower and gem essences for better health on the physical, mental, emotional, and spiritual levels. Three days of classroom and three days of field work. See Appendix J.

2. **Help! and Homeopathy seminar.** Five days of learning all about how to use homeopathy in emergency and first aid crises. This class is for beginners, parents, or anyone who wants to be ready for any emergency with their family and loved ones. The basics of homeopathy are taught—dosage directions, first aid skills, and how to use all of them in their correct order to save a life. Fifty homeopathic remedies will be discussed for flu, colds, measles, mumps, ear infections, and other childhood acute illnesses.

3. **Beginning Medical Astrology.** For the neophyte as well as the professional astrologer. Learn the basics, from the ground up, of medical astrology by zodiac signs and planets. Learn how aspects play a part in health and illness. The Med-Scan technique, which is 95 percent accurate, will be taught. All attendees will have their own natal chart discussed. Homeopathy, vitamins, minerals, flower and gem essences, herbs, and other alternative healing tools will be intermingled throughout the week. Open to everyone.

4. **Advanced Medical Astrology.** Prerequisite: the Beginning Medical Astrology class. The use of Uranian planets, how to use the 90-degree Cosmobiology dial to look for medical problems, and how to pinpoint potential health problems. Continuation with the finer points of the Med-Scan technique, and disease signatures, such as cancer, diabetes, asthma, osteoporosis, and many more. Homeopathy, vitamins, minerals, flower and gem essences, herbs, and other alternative healing tools will be intermingled throughout the week to help with chronic illnesses.

5. **Energy Medicine seminar**. Learn about our energy system, which directly affects our health. The chakras, their function, definition, and importance, the fields of the aura and how each field affects our health. Energy medicine fields—homeopathy, hands-on healing, paper remedies, long-distance healing, flower and gem essences, and our thought processes. Learning how to heal ourselves from within ourselves using these methodologies.

Appendix I

CARA HELP!

When you need help fast, get CARA Help!

CARA Help! is computer software based on *Help! and Homeopathy*, the book by Eileen Nauman and Gail Derin-Kellogg.

To help with the emergency at hand, CARA Help! asks you a series of questions taken directly from the Signs, Symptoms, and Indicators sections in the book. The software then speeds up the process of determining the best homeopathic remedy to use by automatically matching your responses to the known uses of each remedy.

After CARA Help! has determined the best homeopathic remedies to use, it will also show you the most appropriate emergency medical responses.

Sometimes you may not even know the cause of an emergency. No problem with CARA Help! The questions asked are designed to guide you swiftly toward the right homeopathic remedy and the correct emergency medical response.

CARA Help! is an ideal partner for *Help! and Homeopathy*. When you need help fast—use CARA Help!

CARA Help! is part of the growing family of CARA software products that includes modules for homeopathic repertorisation, searching materia medicas, and comparing remedies. The professional version of CARA has full multimedia facilities, including photographs of remedies in glorious color and even spoken audio files from some of the world's leading homeopaths.

For information and to order CARA Help!

Basil Ziv, RSHom (NA)
13 Sala Drive
Suite 400
Richmond Hill, Ontario
Canada L4C8C3

Tel: (905) 886-1060
Fax: (905) 886-1418
e-mail: basilziv@web.net

Appendix J

FLOWER AND GEM ESSENCE
CONSULTANT TRAINING

THREE LEVELS OF CERTIFICATION TO BECOME A NATURAL
ESSENCE CONSULTANT trained by Eileen Nauman

Level 1: Begin to build a foundation on how to conduct a proving, perform actual field work in obtaining a flower or gem essence, and understand preliminary physiology and anatomy of plants. Emphasis is on energy medicine, our chakras, how to perform an assessment on a person, how it relates to the individual, and the potential flower or gem essence that they might need. Discussion of ten flower/gem essences— their unique abilities as discovered via stage 1 and 2 provings. Two field trips, three days of class. AT-HOME ASSIGNMENT: Perform SIX field essences on a plant of your choice in the locale where you live, and do a stage 1 proving on it every other month (six are expected in one year). Send the information and color photos of it via e-mail or jpegs to Eileen. Or, send the info via e-mail, and the photos by post. This information will then be put into the ongoing data bank—with your name on it. Charge: $500.00. First come, first served. Ten people per class.

Level 2: Energy medicine exploration continued. Develop a deeper understanding of the chakras, the colors, and how they connect with flowers and gemstones. A shamanic technique will be shared as to how to retrieve further information from plants. Understand the foundation of a proving, what it is, and how to be a participant in one. Conduct stage 2 provings as a group and build information about essences. Discuss ten flower/gemstone essences. Learn the art of counseling your client; what to say and do and what not to say and do. Discuss the legal ramifications of your practice; the ins and outs of it. Two field trips, three days of class. AT-HOME ASSIGNMENT: Gather at least five to ten friends to conduct a stage 2 proving on SIX flower or gem essences that Eileen will send to you to 'prove.' This will be done every other month (six times in the year). You will not know in advance what they are. You will collate the information from your circle of provers, and mail it to her via e-mail. You will then be told, afterward, what you proved. This helps build our data base. Charge: $500.00. First come, first served. Ten people per class.

Level 3: Learn how to moderate a proving with 20 provers involved with an essence of Eileen' s choice. How to set it up and run it, how to distill information you receive from the field proving logs. Continue learning the art of counseling. Ten flower/gemstone essences will be reviewed. Work with the Natural Essence Test, which helps a client discern what flower/gem essence they need. Deepen your understanding of the Doctrine of Signature. Stage 2 proving of a number of essences during the week. Two field trips, three days of class. TO GRADUATE AS A CONSULTANT FOR EILEEN YOU MUST DO THE FOLLOWING: Conduct a stage 3 proving with an essence that she will choose for you. When you have accomplished this, and the information is assessed, you will then be recognized as a trained consultant. You will receive a major discount on all Blue Turtle Natural Essences. You will be put on the Internet, on a web page, so people can contact you as a consultant. You will also be in a directory in the back of her Natural Essence Materia Medica and Repertory. You will be sent reports on the latest findings from her ongoing data base. Charge: $500.00. First come, first served. Ten people per class.

Note: It takes years to produce a fine essence consultant. It is not done overnight—rather it builds, layer by layer, with the information and education that you need in order to deal with the complexities of such work in a responsible fashion. Not everyone wants to be a consultant and you are welcome to take the level one seminar only, without doing the 'homework' portions. That choice is yours. You cannot take any advanced levels.

1. If you want to become a consultant, then it is mandatory that you take all three levels and conduct the stage provings in each.

2. Failure to conduct the provings eliminates you from the possibility of becoming a consultant.

3. If you are interested in becoming a consultant, please register your name with Eileen Nauman. E-mail her at: docbones@sedona.net or write to her and ask for the registration form: Blue Turtle Natural Essences, PO Box 2513, Cottonwood, AZ 86326. Classes occur once a year. Write for a yearly schedule of events.

4. A graduate consultant will be listed in the directory of any book put out on the provings of essences (Natural Essence Materia Medica and Repertory volumes), as well as being listed on the Internet.

GLOSSARY

A

ABSCESS: A collection of pus in any part of the body. It is characterized by inflammation, heat, redness, swelling, edema, and eruption of the pus. It can also cause fever and chills. Example: Tooth abscess.

ACRID: Burning sensation. Pungent.

ACTIVATED CHARCOAL: Used as an antidote to certain types of poisoning. Contains India ink, which 20% of people are allergic to. Powdered charcoal that has been treated to increase its powers of absorption.

ADD (Attention Deficit Disorder): Developmentally inappropriate inattention or impulsiveness in a child with or without hyperactivity. See: Hyperactive.

ADVANCED LIFE SUPPORT: Lifesaving emergency procedures performed by trained professionals (paramedics). They use cardiac monitoring, defibrillation, intravenous drugs, and advanced airway management equipment and devices.

AIR HUNGER: A shortness of breath; found in diabetic coma.

ALLERGY REACTION: See: **Anaphylactic Shock**.

ALVEOLI: In the lungs; they are small groups of sacs (like grape clusters) within which the exchange of carbon dioxide with oxygen takes place.

ALZHEIMER'S DISEASE: Known as pre-senile dementia or a deteriorating mental state that occurs in the 40 to 60 year old group. It may take months or years to render the person completely helpless.

AMNESIA: Loss or lack of memory; inability to remember past experiences. Opposite: RETROAMNESIA: Person cannot recall memory just before the accident/injury took place.

ANAPHYLACTIC SHOCK: An allergic reaction to a foreign protein or other substances or a sting/bite of an insect/reptile. This can be an allergic reaction to something eaten or inhaled, or via a bite/sting. See: **Wheal**.

ANEURYSM: An artery swells or enlarges as a result of a weakened arterial wall; it bursts open, like a popped balloon, and there is severe life-threatening bleeding.

ANGINA (Pectoris): Heart disease that is brought on by stress or excitement and relieved by rest or prescription of nitroglycerin pills, patch or spray.

ANTIVENIN: A substance that will counteract the effect of an animal or insect venom, such as a rattlesnake bite, a scorpion sting, or the sting of a honeybee.

ANXIETY ATTACK: A sudden, unexpected sense of dread or fear. The person may or may not know what triggers it. May be stress related. See: **Panic Attack**.

ARRHYTHMIA: An irregular or abnormal heart rhythm.

ARTERY: A tubular vessel that carries blood away from the heart to the various parts of the body. If cut, it spurts bright red blood in pulsating movements. See: **Vein**.

ASPHYXIATION: Suffocation.

ASTHMA: Lung disease. Muscles spasm in the small air passageways of the lung(s) and production of mucus plugs these airways, causing breathing problems. See: **Wheeze**.

AURA: A sensation or feeling that precedes a seizure. See: **Convulsive Seizure**.

B

BAKER'S CYST: A cyst with synovial fluid communicating with the synovial fluid within a joint.

BARBITURATE: A prescription drug that depresses the nervous system. Person may be drowsy looking or peaceful looking after taking it.

BASIC LIFE SUPPORT: Simple life-saving emergency procedures that help a person in breathing or circulatory failure. See: **Advanced Life Support**.

BATTLE'S SIGN: Bruising that occurs to the mastoid process directly behind the ear; seen in major head injuries.

BLOOD POISONING: A general term to indicate the presence of bacteria circulating in the blood stream. See: **Sepsis**.

BLOOD PRESSURE: The amount of pressure the blood exerts against the walls of the arteries.

BRACHIAL ARTERY: Located on the inside of the arm between the elbow and shoulder. It is used as an indirect pressure point to slow or stop bleeding.

BRADYCARDIA: The heart beats very slowly but regularly.

BRONCHI: In the lungs, two main branches off the trachea (windpipe) that lead into the right and left lung. There are three major bronchi that form the right lung (3 lobes) and two for the left lung (2 lobes).

BRONCHITIS: The main passageways of the lungs become irritated. This can be from an acute infection or from irritation, such as smoke.

BROWN RECLUSE SPIDER: A very poisonous spider whose bite can cause necrosis, or dying flesh. It is a brown spider with a violin-shaped mark on its head and thorax.

BURSITIS: Inflammation of the bursa, which is a sac or cavity that contains synovial fluid. It is found around tendons or connecting tissue in the vicinity of a joint. It is usually swollen, red, painful, and tender. It limits the physical motion of the person who has it.

C

CANNULA: A plastic device for supplying oxygen that fits around the head with two openings, one for each nostril of the nose.

CAPILLARY REFILL: The ability to restore blood to the capillary blood vessels of either the toe or fingernail after it has been squeezed out. Used to check the patient's circulatory process. Two seconds for blood to come back into the nail is normal. Anything longer than that implies circulation impairment.

CARBON DIOXIDE: CO_2—an odorless, colorless gas resulting from the oxidation of carbon. It is formed in the tissue of the body and is eliminated by the lungs.

CARBON MONOXIDE: CO—a colorless, poisonous gas that is formed by burning carbons or organic fuels in a scant supply of oxygen. It will cause asphyxiation when combined with blood hemoglobin.

CARDIAC ARREST: The heart stops. It ceases to function.

CAROTID ARTERY PULSE: A position on the upper neck (in toward the centerline of the neck/throat region) where the pulse can be felt close to the skin.

CARPAL TUNNEL SYNDROME: Soreness, tenderness, and weakness in one or both wrists, caused by repetitive, unrelieved motion, such as sitting at a computer keyboard and typing all the time. Pressure is placed on the median nerve.

CENTRAL NERVOUS SYSTEM: The brain and spinal cord; the nerves running off the spinal cord are known as peripheral nerves.

CEREBRAL CONCUSSION: The brain is jarred, which results in disturbance to it, but no physical damage occurs to that tissue.

CEREBROSPINAL FLUID: A fluid that the brain and spinal cord float within. Usually it has a translucent to slightly pinkish tinge to it. Seen coming out of the ears, eyes, nose, or mouth, it indicates a very serious head injury.

CERVICAL VERTEBRAE: The first seven vertebrae of the spinal column. They begin at the back of the skull and move downward.

CHEMICAL BURN: A burn that results from a toxic substance coming into contact with the skin.

CHEYNE-STOKES BREATHING: Breathing increases in rapidity and volume and then gradually subsides and ceases entirely for 5 to 50 seconds, when the person begins to breathe again. Sounds like snoring.

CHILBLAINS: Swelling and inflammation of the fingers, toes, or feet, which is caused by cold, damp weather.

CHRONIC FATIGUE SYNDROME: An illness characterized by low grade fever, swollen lymph glands, incredible fatigue, and mild cognitive dysfunction.

CLAVICLE: The collarbone.

CLONIC: Muscular activity that occurs during a generalized epileptic seizure.

COLIC: Spasmodic pain in the abdomen. Often seen in infants.

COPD: Chronic obstructive pulmonary (lung) disease. A slow process of dilation and disruption of the lung's airways and alveoli that is caused by chronic bronchial obstruction.

COMA: A state of unconsciousness where the person cannot be aroused.

COMPLEX PARTIAL SEIZURE: The person may display automatic behavior such as walking aimlessly, chewing, or fumbling with their clothes. Occurs in a partial epileptic seizure; their consciousness may be clouded.

CONGESTIVE HEART FAILURE: The heart loses its ability to pump or circulate the blood adequately. This occurs, usually, as a result of damage to the heart muscle.

CONJUNCTIVA: The lining on the insides of the eyelids; also coats the front of the eyeball.

CONTUSION: A bruise.

CONVULSIVE SEIZURE: Known as a tonic-clonic seizure or a generalized epileptic seizure.

CORNEA: The transparent layer in front of the pupil and iris of the eye.

CREPITUS: When a bone is broken and is grating against the other end of it; you can hear or feel this grinding sensation.

CROUP: An upper respiratory infectious disease that may cause partial airway obstruction. It is often characterized by a barking cough.

CYANOSIS: A blue color or tint to the skin or to the toe and fingernail beds that results from poor oxygenation of the circulating blood supply. They are not getting sufficient oxygen, so they are said to be cyanotic.

CYSTITIS: Inflammation of the bladder caused by infection. Also known as bladder infection.

D

DEFORMITY: Any twisting out of the natural shape of any body part, as in a broken bone. A distortion of shape caused by an injury.

DEHYDRATION: A loss of water from the tissues of the body.

DENTITION: The number, type, and arrangement of the teeth. The cutting of teeth (as in an infant's first teeth).

DELIRIUM: A mental disturbance that may produce hallucinations or restlessness that usually lasts only a short amount of time. Cerebral excitement.

DERMIS: The second layer of skin (the top one is known as the epidermis). The dermis contains nerve endings, blood vessels, sweat glands, and hair follicles. The third layer of the skin is known as the subcutaneous layer.

DIABETES: Insulin deficiency marked by the body's inability to metabolize sugar normally.

DIABETIC COMA: Caused by dehydration and acidosis, the person is unconscious in this uncontrolled diabetic state. It takes several days for this to occur and it can be stopped at any time with the administration of glucose.

DILATE: To swell or to widen; such as the pupil of the eye opening and becoming very dark and black looking. Or a blood vessel dilates (opens up) to allow more passage of blood through it.

DIRECT PRESSURE: Placing the palm of your hand directly over a bleeding wound and pressing on the area enough to either slow or halt the bleeding. Make sure you have put gloves on to protect yourself.

DISLOCATION: The joints are no longer in contact with one another.

DIZZINESS: A sensation of whirling or the feeling that one is going to fall. This is different from vertigo—the two are often confused. See: **Vertigo**.

DYSPHAGIA: Difficulty swallowing.

DYSPHASIA: Difficulty speaking.

DYSPNEA: Difficulty breathing. Shortness of breath.

E

ECCHYMOSIS: A bruise.

ECTOPIC PREGNANCY: A pregnancy where the fetus develops outside the uterus or womb; usually in the Fallopian tube.

EDEMA: Swelling of tissue. Swollen fingers. Swollen ankles, as an example. Also known as 'dropsy.'

EMPHYSEMA: Lung disease where there is extreme dilation and destruction of the alveoli. There is also a poor exchange of oxygen and carbon dioxide. This is also known as COPD, chronic obstructive pulmonary disease.

ENVENOMATION: Injection of venom by an insect or reptile.

EPIGLOTTITIS: A highly dangerous infection that causes swelling of the epiglottis (the flap opening to the trachea) down in the throat.

EPILEPSY: See: **Convulsive Seizure**.

EPPIE SHOT: A syringe of epinephrine used by people with severe allergies. They usually carry this with them and give it to themselves if they have an allergic or anaphylactic reaction.

EPISTAXIS: A nosebleed.

ESOPHAGEAL SPASM: A spasm or constriction in the esophagus. Can be life threatening.

ESOPHAGITIS: Inflammation of the esophagus.

EVISCERATION: A disembowelment; displaced organs outside the body. "Guts hanging out."

EXPIRATION: Exhaling or breathing out air from the lungs. Opposite function is known as inspiration or inhalation.

F

FAINTING: Psychogenic shock caused from excitement or news (good or bad). A temporary loss of consciousness, very brief and not serious.

FEBRILE: A fever.

FEBRILE CONVULSION: During a high fever, usually in children, this is a short seizure that is not dangerous.

FEMORAL ARTERY: The principal artery of the thigh, which supplies blood to the lower abdomen and legs. It is used as an indirect pressure point to slow or halt bleeding in these areas of the body if direct pressure is impossible or does not work. See: **Brachial Artery**, the other indirect pressure point.

FIBROMYALGIA: Pain in the fibrous tissue, muscles, tendons, and ligaments, or other white connective tissue. Occurs mainly in women. There may be stiffness, pain, and aching in specific areas of the body.

FIFTEEN-SECOND GLOBAL: A term used by EMTs to check the ABCs: A—airway (is it open and unobstructed?) B—breathing. Are they? C—circulation. Check pulse. (See: **Pulse**.) A basic examination of an injured person. The airway is not open (blocked by blood, tooth, dentures, food, debris) or they are not breathing, then CPR and/or the Heimlich maneuver must be performed.

FLAIL CHEST (**stoved-in chest**): A blunt injury where three or more ribs are broken in two or more places. They are detached from the rest of the ribcage. When the person inhales, instead of moving out with the rest of the ribs, this section moves inward. This is known as paradoxical motion. These broken ribs can lacerate the lungs or heart.

FLASHOVER: Lightning current travels over the surface of the person on its way to the ground. It is usually experienced as a violent explosion.

FLOATERS: Translucent specks in the eye that float across the eyeball. Protein or cells floating around in the fluid of the eyeball.

FRACTURE: A break in the continuity of a bone; a broken bone.

FROSTBITE: Damage to exposed tissue in cold weather. Skin and deeper tissue are frozen. A serious injury.

FROSTNIP: Cold exposure to the skin, but deeper tissue is not affected.

G

GANGRENE: Death of cells and skin tissue due to loss of blood supply into that area.

GLUCOSE: One of the basic forms of sugar that the body needs to stay alive.

GOUT: Excessive uric acid in the blood that causes arthritis and inflammation of the joints.

H

HARD PALATE: The bony plate that forms the top part of the mouth. The soft palate is composed of mucous membrane and muscles that extend down the throat and hold the food while it is chewed and swallowed.

HEAD-TILT/CHIN-LIFT MANEUVER: Open the airway by tilting the person's head backward and lifting the chin forward, bringing the entire lower jaw forward.

HEAT EXHAUSTION: When a person loses too much water and electrolytes from heavy sweating.

HEAT STROKE: A life-threatening condition caused by exposure to excessive heat (either natural or artificial) that is marked by headache, nausea, dry skin, and muscle cramps.

HEMOPHILIA: A genetic disease where a person inherits the tendency to bleed abnormally. The blood does not clot properly.

HEMOPTYSIS: Coughing up blood or sputum that is tinged with blood.

HEMORRHAGE: Severe bleeding. Bright red spurting blood means an artery is involved. Dark, slower flowing blood means a vein is involved.

HUMIDIFICATION: Adding moisture artificially to a person's mucous membrane surfaces.

HYPERACTIVE: Increased or excessive activity in a child or an adult. Some symptoms are impulsiveness, inability to concentrate, aggressive behavior, constant overactivity, and restlessness. May be due to organic brain damage or symptomatic of a behavior disorder. See: **ADD**.

HYPERTENSION: High blood pressure.

HYPERVENTILATION: A person is taking rapid, deep breaths.

HYPHEMA: There is bleeding within the eyeball itself and it will turn a blood red color as a result. It will obscure the iris or colored portion of the eye.

HYPOTENSION: Low blood pressure.

HYPOTHERMIA: The core temperature within the person's body falls below 95 degrees F after being exposed to prolonged cold and freezing conditions.

HYPOVOLEMIA: A drop (sometimes dramatic) in the circulating blood or other body fluids. See: **Shock**.

HYPOXIA: Oxygen deficient.

I

INCONTINENCE: Involuntary emptying of the bladder or bowels; urination when sneezing or coughing, as an example.

INFARCTION: The death of tissue, which is usually caused by interruption of the blood supply. Seen in a heart attack or myocardial infarction.

INHALATION: Drawing a breath into the body; breathing in. Also known as inspiration. The opposite is exhalation or expiration.

INSULIN SHOCK: A life-threatening situation at times. It comes on suddenly and is due to not eating after a routine dose of insulin or the result of extensive exercise and forgetting to eat on time. Can also occur in hypoglycemic people when they do not eat on time.

IPECAC: See: **Syrup of Ipecac**.

J

JAW-THRUST MANEUVER: Creating an opening in the airway by pulling the person's jaw forward and then pulling the lower lip down.

JOINT: A place where the bones make contact.

K

KUSSMAUL RESPIRATION: Air hunger that manifests as deep sighs of breath.

L

LACERATION: A cut that may have jagged or smooth edges to it. It can be near the surface of the skin or can involve deep muscle tissue, blood vessels, and nerves, as well.

LARYNGOSPASM: The vocal cords in the throat become severely constricted.

LIGAMENT: Fibrous tissue that connects bones to bones. Its job is to give support and strength to the joints.

LOCOMOTOR ATAXIA: Lack of muscle coordination.

LOG ROLL: This maneuver is used in a spinal injury when the person must be moved. It requires two to three people. The person holding the neck and head immobile will count to three and the person is firmly but gently moved from their back onto their side. The second person should concentrate their pull on the heavier portions of the injured person's body—the hips and shoulder region. The person supporting the head cannot do any pushing/pulling—their job is to keep that potential spinal cord injury and neck as immobile as possible, and keep it from moving around at all costs.

LUMBAR: The lower part of the back in which there are five vertebrae; often called the "small" of the back.

M

MANIC DEPRESSION: The person experiences episodes of great mood elevation, restlessness, activity, excitability, or intensity and then sinks into a depression, only to cycle up into the manic behavior once again. The moods alternate.

MODIFIED JAW THRUST: A technique using the index and long fingers to thrust the jaw forward while compressing the patient's nose with your thumbs. If cervical (neck) spinal injury is suspected, keep the head and neck in a neutral position and do not tilt or lift the head.

MYOCARDIAL INFARCTION: A heart attack.

N

NARCOLEPSY: A chronic condition in which the person experiences attacks of drowsiness and sleep. It can happen at any time, driving a car, walking, etc., and not necessarily in bed at night. They cannot control this condition, but are easily reawakened.

NASAL CANNULA: A device that is placed into the nostrils to deliver oxygen.

NECROSIS: Destruction and death of tissues and cells. See: **Gangrene**.

NEURALGIA: Sharp and severe pain along the course of a nerve.

NEUROGENIC SHOCK: Circulatory failure that is caused by paralysis from a spinal cord injury. The nerves to that region (down below the injury) are paralyzed and the blood vessels dilate in response.

NITROGLYCERIN: A drug used in treating angina pectoris. It relaxes the vascular muscles and allows increased blood flow and oxygen to get to the heart muscle.

O

OCCIPUT: The back portion of the head or skull.

OCCLUSIVE DRESSING: A dressing or bandage that closes over a wound and protects it from the air—as in an open chest injury or evisceration (organs hanging out of abdominal area, as an example.) Foil can be used in "sucking chest wounds" as well as in an evisceration—just make sure that the four sides are taped to uninjured skin. Leave a 2-inch opening at the bottom in a sucking chest wound so that air can get in; do not do this for an evisceration.

OSTEOPOROSIS: The bones become porous with age; therefore, they will break more easily. Found especially in women after menopause.

P

PALPATE: To feel or examine by touch. An example: Palpate for the vital signs (pulse, respiration, blood pressure, and temperature).

PALPITATIONS: Rapid, violent, or throbbing pulse. Or abnormal throbbing or fluttering of the heartbeat.

PANCREATITIS: Inflamed condition of the pancreas.

PANIC ATTACK: A sudden, completely overwhelming fear or fright without cause. See: **Anxiety Attack**.

PARANOIA: A psychotic state in which the person may be suspicious, jealous, or brooding in nature, or have fixed ideas or delusions of persecution. These are some of the major symptoms of this disease.

PARIETAL: The walls or sides of the head (not the temple area, but above it). Also pertains to the walls of a cavity.

PEDAL (FOOT) EDEMA: Swelling of the feet or ankles—usually seen in congestive heart failure.

PERFUSION: The process of blood giving nutrients and oxygen and taking carbon dioxide and other toxins or waste material from the tissue and organs. See: **Shock**.

PERIPHERAL NERVOUS SYSTEM: The nerves coming off the spinal cord. There are 31 pairs of spinal nerves and 12 pairs of cranial nerves. They can be sensory nerves or motor nerves.

PERTUSSIS: Whooping cough. An acute, infectious disease with nonstop coughing that ends in a 'whooping' sound upon inhalation of a breath.

PHARYNGITIS: Inflammation at the back of the throat. A sore throat.

PHARYNX: The throat or the area in back of the nose and mouth.

PHLEBITIS: An inflamed vein.

PLAGUE: A disease caused by *Yersina pestis* infection that killed millions in Europe during the 14th century. Characterized by mental confusion, delirium, high fever, restlessness, staggering gait, shock, and finally coma and death.

PLEURISY: The pleura (around the lungs and coating the thoracic cavity) becomes inflamed.

PNEUMONIA: Infection of the lung tissue.

POINT OF TENDERNESS: Placing the index finger gently into the skin to look for tenderness that would indicate injury.

PREMENSTRUAL SYNDROME (PMS): Caused by hormone fluctuation in a woman before her menstrual period. Can include mood alterations, swelling of hands, feet or abdomen, headache, fainting, vertigo, numbness in fingers and toes, backache, bloating and constipation, to name just a few of the symptoms associated with this condition.

PRESSURE POINT: An area where blood vessels run near the bone and if pressure is applied to that area, it can stop bleeding. See: **Brachial** and **Femoral**.

PRIMARY SURVEY: Upon arrival to a scene, there is a primary and secondary survey of the injured person. The primary survey is designed to identify life-threatening conditions. This includes the ABCs and D: Airway—try to rouse the person. If they do not respond, "Look, listen and feel" for breathing. Does the person have an adequate airway? If not, start airway management (CPR). Breathing—is the person having difficulty breathing? Is the breathing shallow, deep, rapid, normal? Are they choking? Is the person's skin turning blue around their mouth or their nailbed (cyanosis)? Circulation—with one hand check the radial pulse on the underside of the wrist below the thumb. If absent in both wrists, place two fingers gently against the carotid pulse in the neck. If both are absent, perform CPR. If pulse is present, assess the person's skin color, temperature, and moisture (perspiration or lack of it). Perform a Capillary Refill on thumbnail to see if there are diminished signs of circulation (if cap refill takes more than 2 seconds to return to healthy pink color on fingernail, there is impairment). Disability—check the person's level of consciousness. Are they alert? If not alert, are they responsive to your voice? If not, are they responsive to pain by rubbing your knuckles up and down on their sternum (breastbone)? Or are they completely unresponsive? See: **Secondary Survey, Capillary Refill**.

PULMONARY EDEMA: Fluid buildup in the lungs that will result in congestive heart failure.

PULMONARY EMBOLISM: A blood clot breaks off from a large vein and travels to the lung.

PULSE: A pressure wave that is felt when the heart contracts and propels blood through the arteries. Key areas to feel for the pulse are the carotid pulse, located in the neck, and the radial pulse, on the wrist. In infants, look for the brachial artery pulse, which is under the upper arm. There are many types of pulse. **Accelerated**: more beats per minute than normal. **Bounding**: pulse reaches higher level, then disappears quickly. **Full**: a distended pulse giving a tense feeling. **Intermittent**: pulse skips a beat. **Irregular**: pulse with a variation of force and frequency. **Soft**: Pulse may be stopped by finger compression. **Thready**: a fine, scarcely perceptible pulse.

PULSE POINT: A place where the artery lies close to the surface of the skin, such as the carotid artery (neck) and the inside of the wrist or the radial pulse.

PULSE RATE: The rate at which the heart is contracting. For adults, 60 to 80 per minute. For a child, 80 to 100 beats per minute.

PUMP FAILURE: When the heart fails to generate sufficient energy to move blood through the body. See: **Shock**.

R

RADIAL ARTERY PULSE: The pulse can be felt on the inside of the wrist, down below the thumb region. The radial artery is very close to the surface of the skin and is an excellent place to feel one's pulse.

RALES: A cracking or rattling breath sound from fluid in the lungs.

RESPIRATION: Breathing.

RESPIRATORY SHOCK: Shock caused by an insufficient amount of oxygen; not enough is being inhaled.

RESTLESS LEG SYNDROME: Intolerable sensations of creeping and internal itching that occurs in the lower legs. Usually worse at the end of a day. Person is constantly moving their legs to seek relief from these sensations.

RHEUMATIC HEART DISEASE: Damage done to the heart due to contracting Rheumatic Fever, a systemic, acute infection.

RHEUMATISM: A general term to denote sore or stiff muscles and joint pain. Includes arthritis.

RHONCHI: Very coarse breath sounds heard in the lungs—usually seen in chronic obstructive pulmonary disease (COPD), emphysema.

S

SALINE SOLUTION: A solution of 0.9% sodium chloride (salt) and distilled water.

SCHIZOPHRENIA: A group of mental disorders. There are four types: simple, paranoid, catatonic, and hebephrenic. Altering of reality, mood changes, inappropriate emotional responses, withdrawn nature, and regressive or bizarre behavior are some of the many symptoms of this complex disease.

SCLERA: The white surface of the eyeball.

SCOLIOSIS: Curvature of the spine. Usually consists of two curves—the original one and then another, which compensates for it.

SECOND DEGREE BURNS: Burns that injure the first two layers of the skin, the epidermis and dermis. Blisters form with this type of burn.

SECONDARY EXAMINATION: After the primary survey is completed, the injured person is examined from head to toe (literally). Both front and back examination. You are looking for wounds, deformities, and points of tenderness, and observing if the person feels pain or any other sensation. See: **Primary Examination**.

SEIZURE: Known also as a convulsion. A general, uncoordinated muscular activity usually associated with loss of consciousness.

SEPSIS: Blood poisoning—very serious, sometimes life threatening. See: **Blood Poisoning**.

SEPTIC SHOCK: Shock caused by infection that damages the walls of the blood vessels.

SHINGLES: Another word for herpes zoster. Herpetic skin eruptions that can occur anywhere on the body. Pain is usually severe after the eruption.

SHOCK: A condition of sudden circulatory failure that causes inadequate (and progressive) perfusion. See: **Perfusion**.

SHOCK POSITION: Lying on the back with elevated legs; keep them warm. The blood will drain out of the enlarged blood vessels in the legs and return to the upper body and heart area for active circulation.

SIDE FLASH: Lightning strikes near a person and 'splashes' through the air onto that individual.

SIGN: Something you observe about the injured person, such as a deformity, bleeding, or hearing wheezing when they breathe.

SIMPLE PARTIAL SEIZURE: A partial epileptic seizure that is limited to one or more extremities, or one side of the body.

SINUSITIS: Inflammation of the sinuses that may include sinus mucus discharge, headache, fever, chills, and pain in the sinus cavities.

SPLINT: A rigid or flexible appliance or material (sticks, a pillow, etc.) to protect and keep the injured part in place and immobile.

SPRAIN: A joint injury in which one of the supporting ligaments is damaged.

STEP-OUTS: A term applied during the physical examination of an injured person. As you run your fingers, beginning at the base of the skull, downward, you are feeling and looking for a 'step-out'—a vertebra that is out of spinal alignment. This is indicative of a potential spinal cord injury and must be treated accordingly.

STERNUM: The breastbone.

STETHOSCOPE: An instrument to listen to sounds within the body, such as heartbeat, lung sound, bowel sound, and blood flow sounds.

STRABISMUS: A deviation of the eyes. The squinting eye will deviate when the other eye is carried in a different direction. The eyes do not follow, as a pair, toward the object looked at. The muscles make the eye squint. It can affect either eye or both of them. Cross-eyed.

STRAIN: A muscle that is torn, overexerted, stretched, or pulled.

STRIDE POTENTIAL: Lightning hits the ground near a person and travels up one leg, down and out the other leg, and into the ground.

STRIDOR: A high-pitched, harsh breathing sound upon inhalation that is often heard in acute laryngeal obstruction.

STROKE: Loss of brain function that is usually due to a cerebral vascular accident.

SUBCUTANEOUS: Under the skin; the third layer of skin, which consists of fat and serves as an insulator for the body.

SUBDURAL: Beneath the dura or cover around the brain and outside the brain itself.

SUBDURAL HEMATOMA: A collection of blood beneath the dura mater and outside the brain.

SUN STROKE: See: **Heat Stroke**.

SUPINE: Lying on the back.

SUPPURATION: The formation of pus.

SWATHE: A bandage that passes around the chest to secure an injured arm to the chest to keep it immobile (the arm is already in a sling).

SYMPTOM: Something the injured person tells you, such as "I feel like I'm going to vomit," or "I'm dizzy," or "I can't breathe."

SYNCOPE: Fainting.

SYRUP OF IPECAC: Preparation of the dried roots of a shrub found in Brazil and other parts of South America. It promotes and causes vomiting and is used to empty the stomach in certain types of poisoning.

T

TACHYCARDIA: Rapid but regular heartbeat or rhythm.

TACHYPNEA: Rapid, excessive shallow breathing.

TENDERNESS: Abnormal sensitivity to touch or pressure that is indicative of a possible injury.

TENDONITIS: Inflammation of a tendon in the body; usually thought of in the Achilles' heel region, the elbow, or the shoulder joint region. Very painful on motion, with inflammation and swelling. Occurs from too much strain placed on the tendon.

THERMAL BURN: A burn caused by heat.

THIRD DEGREE BURNS: A burn that extends into the third layer of the skin—the subcutaneous layer or beyond, into the muscle itself. Skin is usually leathery looking, and white fatty deposits may be visible.

THORACIC VERTEBRAE: The 12 vertebrae attached to the 12 ribs; the upper and middle part of the back or spinal column.

THROMBOSIS: Formation of a blood clot in a blood vessel.

TINNITUS: Ringing sounds in the ear.

TONGUE-JAW-LIFT MANEUVER: Opening the person's mouth by grasping the tongue and lower jaw between the thumb and fingers and lifting them forward.

TONIC-CLONIC SEIZURE: A general epileptic seizure involving most of the brain. Also known as a convulsive seizure.

TONIC-MUSCULAR CONTRACTIONS: A generalized epileptic seizure where there are sustained, rigid, muscular contractions that cause odd, distorted body posturing.

TOURNIQUET: An instrument that compresses the blood vessel to slow or halt bleeding. It should be used only as the last resort.

TRACHEA: The windpipe.

U

URTICARIA: Itching, burning of the skin with many raised, reddened areas. Seen in hives or allergy/anaphylactic reactions.

UVULA: The small, soft structure hanging down from the soft palate at the back of the throat and at the root or base of the tongue.

V

VARICOSE VEINS: Veins, usually in the legs, become twisted, knotted, swollen, and distended. Very painful; can occur anywhere in the body.

VEIN: A tubular-shaped vessel that carries blood FROM the capillaries back to the heart. Blood is slow flowing, a dark red color. See: **Artery**.

VENOM: A poison that is secreted by an animal or insect and injected into the bite/sting.

VENOUS STASIS: The stagnation or slowing of vein circulation of blood in the fingers or toes.

VERTEBRAE: The 33 bones of the spine. There are 7 cervical, 12 thoracic, 5 lumbar, 5 sacral and 4 coccygeal vertebrae in the spine.

VERTIGO: A sensation that things (a room) are moving around in space or objects are moving around the person. Equilibrium is affected as this occurs. Often misdiagnosed as dizziness, but it is not. See: **Dizziness**.

VITAL SIGNS: Signs of life. A person's pulse, respiration/breathing, blood pressure, and temperature.

VOMITUS: Vomited material.

W

WHEAL: A raised, whitish looking area of the skin resulting from a bite of an insect or an allergic reaction to something eaten or inhaled.

WHEEZE: A whistling breath sound, high-pitched and heard on exhalation or release of the breath. Seen in asthmatic people. See: **Asthma**.

X

XIPHOID PROCESS: The lowest part of the sternum or breastbone. It consists of cartilage and can be damaged or torn when performing CPR incorrectly. If torn it can lacerate the liver, injuring the person further.

BIBLIOGRAPHY

Berkow, R., MD. Editor-in-Chief. *The Merck Manual of Diagnosis and Therapy, 16th Edition*. Rahway, NJ: Merck & Co., Inc., 1992.

Boericke, W. MD. *Pocket Manual of Homeopathic Materia Medica*. Philadelphia, PA: Boericke & Runyon Publishers, 1927.

Clarke, J.H., MD. *A Dictionary of Practical Materia Medica*. New Delhi, India: B. Jain Publishers Pvt. Ltd., 1984.

Griffith, H.W., MD. *Complete Guide to Symptoms, Illness & Surgery*. New York, NY: The Body Press/Perigee, 1995.

Heckman, J.D., MD. *Emergency Care and Transportation, 5th Edition*. Rosemont, IL: American Academy of Orthopaedic Surgeons, Revised 1993.

Krupp M.A., MD, and Chatton, M.J., MD, Editors. *Current Medical Diagnosis & Treatment*. Los Altos, CA: Lange Medical Publications, 1982.

Lockie, A., MD. *The Family Guide to Homeopathy*. New York, NY: Fireside Book, 1993.

Manhoff, D. *Outdoor Emergency Medical Guide*. St. Louis, MO: Mosby Year Book, Inc., 1996.

Morrison, R., MD. *Desktop Guide to Keynotes and Confirmatory Symptoms*. Albany, CA: Hahnemann Clinic Publishing, 1993.

Murphy, R., ND. *Lotus Materia Medica*. Pagosa Springs, CO: Lotus Star Academy, 1995.

Thomas, C.L., MD. *Taber's Cyclopedic Medical Dictionary, 13th Edition*. Philadelphia, PA: F.A. Davis Company, 1977.

Vithoulkas, G. *Materia Medica Viva, Volume 1*. Mill Valley, CA: Health and Habitat, Publishers, 1992.

INDEX

INDEX